STUD

The Male Enhancement Guide for Peak Sexual Performance

KIA MICHEL, MD
Beverly Hills Urologist to the Stars
with TONY ALLEMON PA-C

Disclaimer

This book is intended as a reference volume only and is not a medical manual. The information given here is designed to help you make informed decisions about your health with the help of a qualified healthcare provider. It is not intended as a substitute for any treatment that may have been prescribed by your doctor. If you suspect that you have a medical problem, please seek a competent medical practitioner, such as a board-certified urologist or your primary care provider.

Any mention of specific brand names, companies, organizations, or authorities in this book does not imply endorsement by the author or publisher, nor does mention of specific companies, organizations, or authorities imply that they endorse this book, its author, or the publisher. Any mention of active clinical trials is not an endorsement of that particular therapy, nor a definitive statement on its efficacy or safety. Rather, active clinical trials are mentioned to inform the reader that these studies exist. Please contact the study organizer or your qualified healthcare provider to learn more about the eligibility criteria of clinical trials.

Internet addresses, website URLs, and phone numbers given in this book were accurate at the time it went to press. For the most up-to-date information, please visit us at comprehensive-urology.com. There, you can also find the bios of our board-certified urologists and physician assistants who can provide you with their expert opinions on your best course of treatment.

TABLE OF CONTENTS

REDEFINING OPTIMAL SEXUAL HEALTH

Sexual function is crucial to a man's self-esteem and identity. More men are interested in preserving and optimizing their sexual function, regardless of age. Today, many men are recognizing their sexual dysfunction and limitations and are openly seeking ways to improve their sexual health.

Historically, erectile dysfunction was viewed as simply a lack of blood flow to the penis. However, over the past several decades, our understanding has evolved. We now recognize the nuances that contribute to stronger erections and enhanced sexual performance. A key component in diagnosing and treating erectile dysfunction is understanding that it can be a multifactorial issue. Factors such as cardiovascular health, neurological health, hormonal balance, pelvic floor tone, and psychological well-being all play a role in optimizing a man's sexual health and functionality.

In this book, we share key points for men to consider in their journey toward sexual self-improvement and optimization. It has been rewarding to see more men naturally optimize their sexual function and reduce their dependence on medications. Witnessing the transformation of a man from insecure or unable to confident and sexually proficient is incredible. With advancements in medical technology, nearly any man, at any age, can achieve great sexual function.

Let's explore the many non-invasive approaches to optimizing your sexual performance. After I explain each of the therapies, I will introduce you to the STUD Protocol for optimized sexual performance that I use with my patients at my Beverly Hills clinic, Comprehensive Urology.

If you've found your way to this book, see it as a call to action to recover your vitality and full exuberance. The goal is simple. When you look in the mirror, you will see your inner stud. And others will see it too.

REDEFINING OPTIMAL SEXUAL HEALTH

At the heart of a man's confidence is his ability to perform sexually.

Regaining sexual function and gaining confidence are interlinked. When we work with our patients, I want to get to the core of the matter. Part of regaining that confidence comes with a man being able to trust his body again. By being able to rise to the occasion when it's time to engage, a man feels his inner stud again.

Medications can be very helpful for treating erectile dysfunction, however, I want my patients to be able to achieve satisfying erections and orgasms without being dependent on daily treatment. There are other ways to address circulatory issues that impact their ability to have erections. For instance, many of my patients who use periodic Shockwave Therapy and begin exercising regularly don't need Viagra or Cialis. With all the advances in technology, we not only have the means to address sexual dysfunction, rather we can go beyond your baseline and optimize your sexual performance.

While I value the medical interventions at my disposal to treat sexual and urological issues, I think of these therapies as part of a longer journey towards optimized sexual health. Think of your sexual health as three layers of a pyramid. From the bottom to the top, we have the following layers:

- Recovery of Sexual Function
- Anti-Aging and Sexual Rejuvenation
- Sexual Optimization

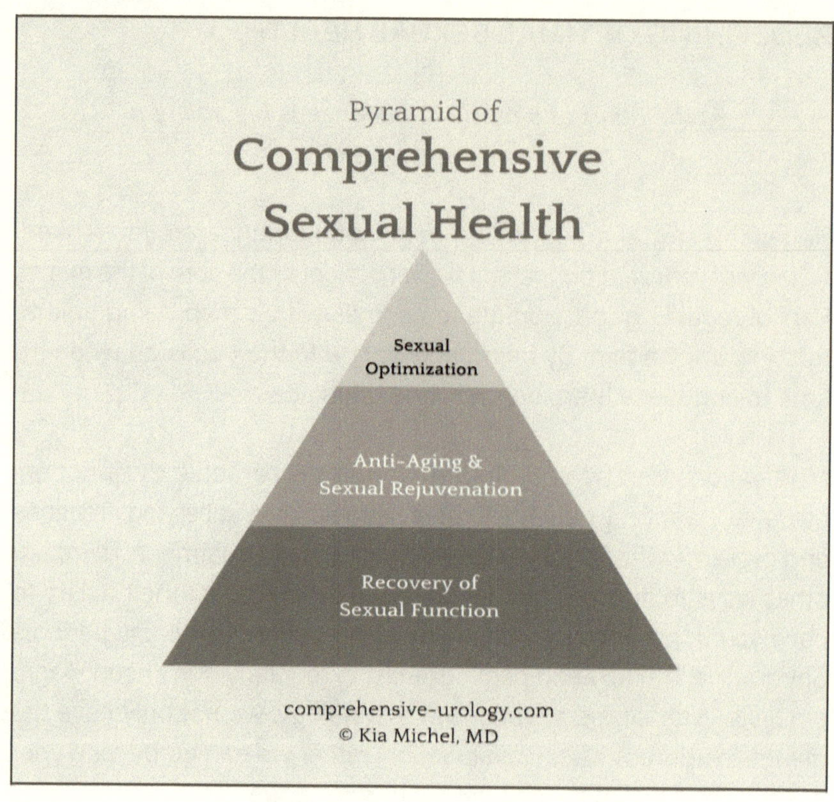

Diagram 1: *Pyramid of Comprehensive Sexual Health*

I share this pyramid of comprehensive sexual health to help you break out of the mindset that you wait until something is broken until you ask someone for help to fix it. This outdated mentality is passive and contributes to the gradual decline of your vitality and sexual vibrancy as you age. Don't fall into that slow, downward slide. Be active with your sexual health. Take action to not only preserve your libido and sexual function, but to maximize it beyond your self-imposed limits. There is a resignation in the statement "I'm getting old" that surrenders responsibility for your sexual health and youthful exuberance. Instead, say "don't let the old man in."

Dear reader, be the member of your social circles who exudes that spark of life. It begins by taking responsibility for your vitality. The first step is reframing how you look at your sexual health beyond disease and sexual dysfunction. Let me explain the levels of the pyramid of comprehensive sexual health.

Recovery of Sexual Function:

This is the foundational level of your sexual health that focuses on addressing the medical conditions that interrupt your ability to have a satisfying sex life. Circulatory issues, hormone imbalances, benign prostate growth as seen in BPH, or prostate cancer must be addressed to have your overall health and a healthy sex life.

Anti-Aging & Sexual Rejuvenation:

New technologies and medical interventions have extended the longevity of our sexual vitality and overall physical health. The problem is most people are stuck in the "if it ain't broke, don't fix it mentality" and don't realize that they can be doing so much more to preserve and enhance their sexual satisfaction. Hormone replacement therapy, lifestyle changes, Shockwave Therapy for penile rejuvenation and ThermiVa for vaginal rejuvenation are all great options to extend your youthful nature.

Sexual Optimization:

At the top of the pyramid, we reach sexual optimization where you can actually achieve new levels of sexual performance and satisfaction during intercourse. Sexual optimization means reaching your full erections with consistency and enhancing the size and condition of your genitals. This includes Platelet-Rich Plasma (PRP) penile injections, Botox penile injections, and Scrotox injections (Botox for your scrotum) which are often combined with Shockwave Therapy for penile rejuvenation.

During sexual optimization treatments with our heterosexual couples, I often recommend that the women partner try ThermiVa vaginal rejuvenation at the same time to optimize the pleasure of both partners. For our gay couples, mutual sexual optimization using the same therapies can bring a new spark to your relationships. Doing the journey together is fun while increasing intimacy and mutual support.

BENEFITS OF OPTIMIZED SEXUAL HEALTH:

- Improved personal confidence
- Increased ability to connect with others
- Improved intimacy in relationships
- Increased happiness
- Enhanced vitality and longevity

The quality of your treatment is only as good as the quality of your doctor. Too many of us just accept the decline of our physical vitality without knowing the various options that are available to recover it. Customized treatment plans can help you rejuvenate your libido and restore your sexual health. But this is also an opportunity to do the inner work. It starts by looking in the mirror and remembering your inner stud, that sexual being that connects with confidence. When your libido and mood begin to rise from successful sexual health treatments, you'll notice that glow around you in the bathroom mirror. You'll be surrounded by an air of confidence. You'll see your inner stud. And others will see it too.

YOU DON'T NEED TO AGE PREMATURELY

Unfortunately, so many of us are aging prematurely when considering how far modern sexual medicine has come. Don't be passive and slide into the resignation of "getting old" prematurely. There is so much that you can do. If you are a younger man who maybe has had their first experience of having an enlarged prostate or erectile issues, take comfort in knowing that early intervention will ensure that you have a very long and satisfying sex life.

As you read this guidebook, I want you to remember this pyramid to help you step outside of the box that society has conditioned you to believe. You are most likely carrying some self-imposed limitations that will be validated by your friends, colleagues, and cohorts. Recognize how you limit your own potential. Be aware of your limiting beliefs about what you are able to experience in your intimate relationships. There are more ways to achieve optimal sexual health today than ever before. That means increased libido, more frequent sex, more enjoyable sex, with reliable sexual performance.

At the end of the book, I share the details of the Stud Protocol that we use at Comprehensive Urology in Beverly Hills, Los Angeles to rejuvenate the sexual organs of men. It includes male enhancement options to increase endowment, stamina, and reliability of erections.

Take the Stud Protocol challenge. Give yourself permission to surprise yourself.

PART I

YOUR CONFIDENCE

1. Your Libido, Your Vitality, Your Sustained Youth

What drives me as a physician is seeing the transformation of my patients who recover their optimal sexual health and vitality. Sexual health conditions not only interrupt the normal function of the body, but also can weigh on our minds. When men can't engage in the intimacy of intercourse, they lose confidence.

This loss of confidence can hurt their intimate relationships. So many times, I see how a partner feels that they are no longer attractive or wanted because a man shies away from sex without communication. Men tend to suffer in silence, but they don't realize that their partners may be suffering along with them. It's embarrassing for a man to admit that he can't get an erection or to maintain an erection during sex. But the avoidance can damage intimacy in the relationship, especially if the man feels hopeless about aging.

With all of the treatment options and advances in technology that we have today, many men don't realize that they are aging prematurely when they could have many more years of satisfying and invigorating sex. The biggest obstacle to sexual health is not asking for help. The sooner treatment is started, the more favorable the results. This is why I always make sure that my patients feel safe talking about their symptoms.

As you restore trust in your body's ability to consistently perform during sex, your confidence in your sexual ability will grow. But there is also an internal aspect of confidence. When you look in the mirror, you need to be happy with the person you see looking back at you. I encourage you to use your recovery and optimization of your sexual health as the impetus to change your life for the better. Make this phase of your life the most rewarding part yet. It starts by opening up and expressing how you feel about your current state of health, knowing that there are many ways for you to change it. Don't suffer in silence. Ask for help, both from a board-certified urologist and a qualified mental health professional. See this as investing in your self-care and well-being.

Treatment brings hope. My goal isn't just to restore a man's ability to have satisfying intercourse, rather I want my patients to achieve their optimal sexual health. Optimal sexual performance isn't just about resolving symptoms. It's about restoring libido and physical health to such a degree that when that patient looks in the mirror, they exude confidence. When they walk into the room, others immediately notice their vitality.

Part of achieving optimal sexual health is seeing yourself as a confident and capable man.

2. Intimacy: How Sex Brings You Close to Your Partner

Without the confidence to engage in sex, intimacy fades in a couple. When one partner is experiencing erectile dysfunction or reduced libido due to a hormonal or urological issue, the other partner can feel rejected. Very often, the decrease in sexual interest has nothing to do with the desire for their partner. Rather, during foreplay, a man may find that as much as he wants to engage in his mind, his body just isn't responding as it once had.

So many men suffer in silence when they experience erectile dysfunction and low libido. Having low testosterone can feel similar to depression in that there can be suppressed desire, fatigue, a cloudy mind, and an overall lack of enthusiasm. However, the cause of low T is different from clinical depression, as the root cause is a drop in testosterone levels.

Experiencing erectile dysfunction can be embarrassing and disheartening because there's so much stigma around a man's ability to perform sexually. There's peer pressure to have solid erections and to last long enough to satisfy your partner. So many of my patients erroneously believe that if they are experiencing erectile dysfunction, they are somehow failing. But in reality, your body needs help and asking for that help is the first step to resolving it.

Our bodies need maintenance. Our hearts need cardiovascular exercise to function optimally. Our brains need rest in order to think clearly. Why would our penises be any different than the rest of our body?

Intimacy begins with you. It starts by having self-compassion during a challenging moment in your life. When you experience ED or low libido, reassure yourself that it's OK to ask for help in the same way you would if you caught a cold or discovered a heart condition. Your body needs help, and getting the right care is an act of self-care. My patients are always relieved when they discover that they're not alone. They receive hope from the latest, minimally invasive treatments that raise their sexual health. They soon recover their confidence to engage.

Reclaiming your confidence happens when you take responsibility for your vitality and sexual health. This means that when your body is sending you signals that it's struggling, you are responsible for responding. Asking for help is the right thing to do when your body is struggling. If you saw a check engine light come up on your car, you would take the car to the mechanic. Why would you ignore the signals from your more precious vehicle that is your body? It's the only one you've got!

As you regain your vibrant libido and improve your erectile performance, you're ready to engage intimately again with renewed confidence. Your partner will feel more attractive and wanted. You will feel a sense of empowerment knowing that your body is ready to engage.

As they regain their peak sexual performance, many of my patients use this momentum to make other healthy changes in their lives. They start exercising again, which improves their mood, overall health, and endurance. Many lose weight and find that the combination of treatments and lifestyle changes help them recover to a more youthful man when they look in the mirror. See this obstacle in your sex life as an opportunity to transform your life. It all begins with shifting your mind frame around being responsible for your vitality. Once you take ownership for your spark of life and the care of your body, a new wave of youthful energy moves through you.

The first step is to claim responsibility for your health. It begins by seeing a urologist to resolve the physical conditions. It continues each time you look in that mirror and see a vital man staring back at you.

ThermiVa for vaginal rejuvenation and Shockwave Therapy for penile rejuvenation combined offer increased sexual satisfaction and intimacy for heterosexual couples. Gay and lesbian couples can also share the same therapies to increase sexual pleasure and their intimate bond.

FEELING CONFIDENT IN YOUR OVERALL HEALTH

Many patients come to us for a second opinion. Very often, the reason
that a treatment failed one of my new patients seeking a second
opinion is that they were misdiagnosed. It happens regularly.

To ensure that you are getting the best care, here's what your healthcare
professional should check during your sexual health evaluation.

1. Psychological health: many healthcare providers won't ask much
    about your mental well-being. However, this plays a major role
    in sexual health and confidence during intercourse. If you feel
    that your mood is off, you are not sleeping well, or you are overly
    stressed, bring these points up and ask your practitioner for
    guidance. If they don't provide adequate support, seek help from
    additional providers. It's important.

2. Nerves and vessels: ask for a non-invasive evaluation of your
    micro-vessels and micro-nerves which can be easily assessed
    by evaluating your sweat glands through tiny electric impulses.

3. Hormones and metabolism: ask for a full hormone panel and
    metabolic evaluation with your blood work. The blood tests
    should include:
    a. CBC (Complete Blood Count)
    b. Chem 13 Panel
    c. Thyroid Panel
    d. Testosterone Panel (to include Total T, Free T, bioavailable T,
        Sex Hormone Binding Globulin),
    e. DHEA, Estradiol
    f. Vitamin D Levels
    g. Extensive Lipid Panel

Be the advocate of your health and proactively ask your provider for these evaluations.

CONFIDENCE IN YOUR PENIS SIZE

Big Penis Energy is a slang term that refers to the air of confidence a man has when he is satisfied with the size of his penis. Having doubts about your ability to satisfy your partner(s) during sex due to the size of your penis can impact your sexual performance and enjoyment. If you're having doubts about your penis size, talk to your urologist about it.

Does size matter during sex?

Sexual satisfaction isn't necessarily dependent on your penis size. Size is an individual preference between the members of the partnership. In particular, a woman who arrives at orgasm through clitoral stimulation will be more focused on the stimulus happening outside the vagina than the internal sensations. Women more inclined to clitoral orgasms may be fine with an average or slightly smaller penis, as long as they are receiving adequate stimulation externally. The clitoris is a pearl-shaped mound at the top of the labia (vaginal lips) which contains a bundle of sensory nerves.

However, a good amount of women report that they desire a larger sized penis because in order to arrive at an orgasm, they need internal vaginal stimulation. Just as there are women who arrive at orgasm through clitoral stimulation, others need direct friction on their G-Spot, which is usually located internally on the top part of the vagina behind the pubic bone. The G-spot isn't actually an organ, rather it is a network of nerves that extend from the clitoris into the internal tissue of the vagina. If you think of the clitoris as the head of a jellyfish, and the tendrils of the jellyfish being nerves that extend from the clitoris, then the G-spot is the bundle of nerve endings that hang below the clitoris inside the wall of the vagina. Women who need this kind of stimulation to have an orgasm are more likely to prefer men with larger penises because more volume means that there's more surface area to stimulate these sensitive nerves.

There are another group of women that may need even deeper penetration in order to experience an orgasm. For these women, the cervix, which is the opening between the back of the vagina and the uterus where the baby is conceived, needs stimulation. Because the cervix is the furthest area of all the orgasm zones discussed, a longer penis is more likely to be the preference of a woman who needs deeper stimulation to feel the full pleasure of sex.

Just like men, the size and depth of a woman's vagina is individual. So the size of the penis during sex can have an impact based on the size of both genitalia as well as which orgasm zone is principal for the woman. Bottom line: every woman is different, and penis size depends on the couple. Simply asking your partner how they've arrived at orgasm in the past will help build intimacy and confidence during sex.

For gay partners, penis size is also a personal preference. Some gay men prefer more stimulation to their prostate during intercourse, which can produce orgasms. In this case, they would want a partner with more volume. Others desire less prostate stimulation to experience an orgasm. Some gay men prefer only penile stimulation, which isn't size-dependent. Opening up a conversation about preferences during sex, including the taboo topic of penis size, can lead to greater intimacy and satisfaction.

For those of my patients who lack confidence to engage because of inner doubts about penis size, you need not suffer in isolation. There is help to enhance your penis size with minimally invasive therapies such as penile injections and non-invasive Shockwave Therapy. If your doubts about your penis size are interrupting meaningful opportunities for intimacy, there is nothing wrong with seeking the help of a trained therapist. For instance, I've had patients come to me who have the very real diagnosis of micropenis, which is a penis that is significantly smaller than average. Being able to enhance their size has given them the confidence to start dating again. Consulting a qualified urologist or surgeon regarding male enhancement options, such as penis enlargement, can build the confidence you need to find a suitable partner. Please consult a qualified medical practitioner when evaluating the risks and benefits of penis enlargement procedures.

WHAT'S THE AVERAGE PENIS SIZE?

Occasionally, my male patients aren't sure how to have that conversation with their partner about sexual satisfaction, so they ask me as a urologist, "What's the average penis size?" This question is also a popular search term on search engines. Again, a satisfying penis size depends on the personal preferences of your partner. What's right for one partner might not be right for another. Our genetics are our starting point when it comes to our shapes and sizes. Our preferences further inform this conversation that often comes in intimate conversations. At the end of the day, what's important is that you feel happy with your penis and that you can have satisfying intercourse with your partner.

Science has an answer to the penis size question. There have been studies on both the average size of penises as well as penis size in relation to the frequency of orgasms in women.

Average Penis Size: The British Journal of Urology International published a comprehensive review study and found that the average erect penis is 5.16 inches (13.1 cm) in length. Most men fall within an inch or so of this average (between 4–6 inches). Anything over 6 inches (15.2 cm) during an erection is considered a large penis.[1]

The Link Between Penis Size and Orgasm Rates: A study of 323 women titled "Women Who Prefer Longer Penises Are More Likely to Have Vaginal Orgasms" published in the Journal of Sexual Medicine found that a longer penis does enhance vaginal orgasm occurrence, but it didn't necessarily enhance the number of clitoral orgasms. Of the 323 women, 160 said they only experienced vaginal orgasms, meaning they needed internal stimulation during intercourse to have an orgasm. Of these 160 women, 33.8 percent preferred longer-than-average penises (longer than 6 inches (15.2 cm)), 60 percent said size made no difference and 6.3 percent said longer was less pleasurable than shorter.

In this study, the "average penis size" was described as longer than the previous study, with the average being 5.8 inches (14.9 cm) and 6.1 inches (15.5 cm). Anything over 6.1 inches was considered a "longer penis"[2].

Overall, the average penis size is somewhere between 5 and 6 inches when erect. Micropenis, also called hypoplasia of the penis, is defined as being 3.67 inches (9.3 cm) or less when stretched. A micropenis

---

1 Veale, D., et al. (2015). Am I normal? A systematic review and construction of nomograms for flaccid and erect penis length and circumference in up to 15,521 men. British Journal of Urology International, 115(6), 978-986. DOI: 10.1111/bju.13010

2 Costa, R. M., et al. (2012). Women Who Prefer Longer Penises Are More Likely to Have Vaginal Orgasms (But Not Clitoral Orgasms): Implications for an Evolutionary Theory of Vaginal Orgasm. The Journal of Sexual Medicine, 9(12), 3079-3088. DOI: 10.1111/j.1743-6109.2012.02917.x

can function normally and often results from a reduced amount of androgens (masculine hormones) while the fetus develops in the womb. Between 6 and 7 inches (17.8 cm) is considered larger than average and 7+ inches in length is considered a large penis.

While I take my patients' concerns about their penis size seriously, I also remind them that sexual satisfaction and orgasms are influenced by many factors beyond anatomy. Emotional connection, communication, sexual technique, and individual preferences all play substantial roles in a satisfying sex life. These two particular studies alone are not meant to reduce the act of sexual satisfaction to numeric terms. I just believe in giving a straightforward answer to a popular question based on science. What is most important is that you are happy with your size and that you feel confident in your ability to satisfy your partner. If you harbor doubts, the loss of confidence can lead to emotional distancing and avoidance of sex. This can hurt intimacy, so opening up a dialogue with your therapist, urologist, and partner is essential.

Fortunately, there are minimally invasive male enhancement therapies available to explore if therapy alone does not restore your confidence to engage.

PART II

YOUR PENIS

3. A Healthy Penis: Erection, Ejaculation, and Orgasm

Your penis is your friend. Think of all the good times you had together. Your penis is such an important part of your relationship that even some couples give him a nickname.

Sometimes, our friends need help. The problem is that when men have problems with their special friend, they tend to ignore it. Even if you'd drop what you were doing to help a real friend change their flat tire on the side of the road, you might not give your special friend the same level of attention when he needs you most. Why neglect your penis if it's giving you signals that something is wrong?

For many men, that signal comes in the form of a change in their erections. Perhaps the erections happen less often, or they arrive softer than before. Part of having a healthy penis is to get care when something changes, and that means asking your urologist to check things out. Let's start by understanding the normal function of a healthy penis.

Before we go into the diseases and conditions that interrupt a satisfying sex life, I want to share about the elements of a healthy sex life. Each of these elements can be enhanced beyond your everyday experience, even when nothing's wrong. Optimizing your hormone levels not only stops a potential problem before it starts, but it also leads to more libido and zeal in your life. Why wait for erectile dysfunction to arrive when you can experience penile rejuvenation using Shock Therapy to enhance your erections proactively? Before my prostate cancer patients go in for surgery, I have them prehabilitate before the procedure with Shockwave Therapy and penile injections because it raises the bar on what is possible post-op. Begin thinking about your health beyond the baseline accepted by your colleagues, friends, and neighbors. Aim for optimal sexual health.

HEALTHY ERECTIONS

Before we speak about erectile dysfunction, let's discuss what happens during a healthy erection. The penis is a vascular organ, meaning it's made up primarily of a series of blood vessels. There are 2 kinds of blood vessels:

1. Arteries that let fresh blood into the penis from the heart
2. Veins that pull the blood out of the penis, returning to the heart

During an erection, the blood flow to the penis increases, and the arterial blood vessels get engorged which shuts off the veins. By pinching off the veins, the engorged arteries increase the pressure inside the penis, causing it to enlarge and to get hard. Once the blood inflow starts to diminish, the veins are no longer compressed and the blood starts draining from the penis, leading to a loss of erection. So the mechanics of an erection are all about blood flow, which is why your overall cardiovascular health has such a big impact on your ability to have and sustain your erections.

A normal, healthy erection can sustain from anywhere between a few minutes to a couple of hours. The average time of an erection during penile-vaginal intercourse is somewhere between 5–10 minutes long according to studies[3].

An erection sustained beyond 4 hours could be a sign that you have a disease condition called priapism which is harmful to your penis.

---

3   https://pubmed.ncbi.nlm.nih.gov/16422843/

Having the blood flow to your penis shut off beyond 4 hours can lead to cell death because the cells can't get fresh oxygen from new blood. It can also lead to erectile dysfunction if left untreated.

STEPS FOR ACHIEVING AN ERECTION

Step 1: The arousal process begins with psychological or physical stimulation: eyes, ears, touch, and smell activate a response in the brain.

Step 2: The brain begins to trigger messages that travel down the spine and to the pelvic nerves. Also, the brain tells the glands to produce certain hormones such as testosterone and blood chemicals such as nitrous oxide into the bloodstream.

Step 3: The pelvic nerves send a signal to the arteries of the penis to open up and let more blood in. The arteries clamp the veins down to prevent the new blood from leaving the vascular tissue of the growing penis.

Step 4: Blood flow to the penis increases substantially, resulting in a strong erection that doesn't let the blood come out of the vascular tissue.

Step 5: With climax (orgasm) or lack of continued stimulation, the blood flow to the penis decreases as the veins reopen to pull the blood out of the penis towards the heart.

Step 6: The erection subsides.

The erection all begins with that first step of the arousal process that starts with a full sensory experience. The smell of flowers, perfume, and sweat can begin the process. Or perhaps it's the appearance of a partner, the colors they wear, or the beautiful scenery around you. Compliments, foreplay, and flirting are part of the art form that starts the mating process. The psychological stimulation changes your mental state, relaxes your body, and gets you "in the mood." Your penis starts to respond with an erection afterward. So, your brain is actually the organ where the whole sexual process starts.

How do we optimize your mental state for the best erections and sexual experience?

KEY PHYSIOLOGIC ELEMENTS FOR AN OPTIMIZED ERECTION

1. Positive mindset and adequate stress relief
2. Normal testosterone
3. Healthy nerves
4. Healthy vessels
5. Proper stimulation

POSITIVE MIND SET

Many men we see who have erectile dysfunction have a psychological component

to their ED. Their anxiety manifests physically as stress and tension in the body. This releases certain stress hormones such as cortisol and adrenaline which put the body and mind in a fight-or-flight response. To have a satisfying erection and to fully engage in the pleasure of sex, we need to be in a calm, restful state which is the opposite of a fight-or-flight response.

This is why when men go on vacations, their sexual function can often return to normal because they aren't stressed about work. This is also why couples' therapy can help defuse the tension of relationship conflicts that can improve the couple's sex life.

Performance anxiety can hinder erections. Many men are so worried about what their partner may think about their sexual performance, including how their body looks and the size of their penis, they never get into the relaxed state necessary to engage. In this agitated state, the brain never relaxes enough to be able to send the stimulation signals to the penis to get a good, solid erection.

The type of stimulation is a very personal preference. Some men can get erections with only certain types of stimulation (for example oral sex), but not with others (for example, vaginal or anal sex).

So what can we do to consistently have healthy erections?

DR. KIA MICHEL'S CHECKLIST FOR HEALTHY ERECTIONS

1. Check your testosterone level: T can affect your confidence and sense of well-being, and can enhance mood and lower underlying anxiety. For more information, see "Part IV: Your Testosterone."
2. Exercise daily: even 15 minutes of cardio can help with mood optimization through the release of hormones called endorphins.
3. Therapy: getting professional help can make a big difference for your anxiety and self-esteem.
4. Reducing alcohol consumption, cigarette use, and getting help for drug addictions will greatly enhance your sexual performance.

TESTOSTERONE IS CRUCIAL FOR
YOUR SEXUAL HEALTH

Our testosterone levels naturally start declining around age 45 and continue to go down into our 80s. However, there are several ways to preserve a healthy level of testosterone well into your elder years. A quick way to see if you have sufficient testosterone on your own is to observe how many mornings you wake up with an erection without physical stimulation or foreplay. Our testosterone naturally goes up and down in our bloodstream following a predictable cycle. Our resting testosterone level when we first get up is a fair indicator of your testosterone. If you wake up most mornings with an erection, that's a good sign for your testosterone level. However, if you don't wake up often with erections, or you're feeling sluggish with brain fog and a low mood, have your physician do a full hormone panel/metabolic work-up to check your T levels and related hormones.

We'll be extensively covering treatment options for low T in Part IV of the book; however, I'd like to impress upon you the importance of having a healthy testosterone level for enjoying a healthy sex life.

IMPACTS OF A HEALTHY TESTOSTERONE LEVEL

1. Sharper thinking: many men with low T feel that they have mental fog, or can't recall names or information as readily, or they feel like their mind is working more slowly than normal.
2. Balanced mood: many men with low T feel depressed, have increased anxiety, or both. We have treated many men with low T that after their testosterone was normalized they came off of their antidepressants completely and their low T had been initially misdiagnosed as depression.

3.   Improved libido: many men with low T present with a lowered sex drive (libido)—often this can be reversed with testosterone optimization.
4.   Stronger erections: many men with low T who have their testosterone levels optimized, notice that their erections get stronger.
5.   Improved energy: many men with low T feel that they get tired sooner, need to take naps, can't recover as quickly after workouts, or don't have the drive to be as active in general. Once optimized, many men can regain these normal functions and increased states of energy. Increased overall physical activity can improve overall cardiovascular health, including blood flow to the penis.
6.   Improved muscle mass: normal testosterone levels are key for maintaining normal muscle mass and skin appearance. With an active lifestyle, most men can regain muscle mass with testosterone optimization.
7.   Improved bone health: low T can accelerate bone loss in men and can be a risk factor for bone fractures due to osteoporosis.
8.   Improved metabolism: when T levels are normalized, many men notice that their blood sugar levels and lipid profiles (cholesterol and triglyceride levels) improve!
9.   Improved metabolism can improve overall cardiovascular health, including blood flow to the penis.

HEALTHY NERVES AND HEALTHY VESSELS

Unless there has been trauma to the nerves (such as a stroke, surgery, radiation, or physical trauma) nerves typically will function properly unless there are nutritional issues, or microvascular problems. What is microvascular? The blood vessels in the body can be broken up into large vessels, medium-sized vessels, small vessels, and very small vessels (microvascular).

It is the micro-vessels that ultimately carry blood to the cells in each organ as well as to the nerves. One of the earliest signs of microvascular disease is nerve dysfunction. So, cardiovascular health actually leads to improved nerve function as well.

Some key risk factors for cardiovascular disease are:

- Diabetes
- Hypertension
- Obesity
- Imbalanced cholesterol levels
- Inactive lifestyle
- Smoking
- Kidney or liver failure

DR. KIA MICHEL'S CHECKLIST TO PRESERVE CARDIOVASCULAR AND NERVE HEALTH

1. Lead an active lifestyle
2. Perform cardiovascular exercise 3–4 times a week for about 40 minutes
3. Maintain ideal body weight
4. Eat a more plant-based diet: reduce the portion size of meats and increase the veggies to cover half of your plate
5. Get good, quality sleep
6. Avoid toxins including tobacco, too many prescription painkillers, and excessive alcohol consumption

Can you check your nerve and microvascular health? Yes, you can. There are simple non-invasive studies that can assess your microvascular health as well as your micro-nerve health. Just ask your healthcare specialist.

PROPER STIMULATION FOR ERECTIONS

A key component to maintaining a strong erection is sustained physical stimulation of the penis. Some men complain of losing their erections during sex, and on further assessment, their partner is too loose or overly lubricated. Once these issues are addressed, many men realize that they can have normal erections with proper stimulation.

HEALTHY EJACULATION

During an orgasm, the fluids in the prostate and seminal vesicles (structures right next to and connected to the prostate) get repeatedly squeezed out by the muscles in the pelvis that go into repeated contractions. If not much volume is coming out, it could be a sign of multiple issues, including low testosterone level, prostatic enlargement (prostatitis or BPH), pelvic floor dysfunction, or rarely prostate cancer.

So if a man notices that the ejaculatory volume is going down, it's important to get it assessed. If the force of ejaculation is diminished, then treating the underlying conditions can cause significant improvement. Strengthening the pelvic floor and addressing underlying ejaculatory issues can result in shooting a harder stream during an orgasm which can result in more pleasure and may help for couples trying to conceive a child.

What if the man who does not have any ejaculatory dysfunction wants to have stronger and more forceful ejaculations? For such patients, pelvic floor therapy can be effective. With this approach, the pelvic floor muscles are stimulated and strengthened, thereby allowing the contractions to be stronger, resulting in more forceful ejaculations.

AMAZING ORGASMS

Improving the quality of orgasms in men involves both physiological and psychological factors. On the physical end of the equation, a gentleman needs to have consistent and reliable erections. Once this has been established, it's possible to enhance orgasms through regenerative therapies like Shockwave Therapy to further enhance blood flow that brings the hormones and neurotransmitters involved in the orgasm process into the area. Pelvic floor exercises ensure that you are having a full and satisfying ejaculation. By living a healthy lifestyle, your blood vessels and nerves will coordinate beautifully at the climax of your symphony.

HORMONES AND NEUROTRANSMITTERS DURING AN ORGASM

Orgasm in men is not just a physical phenomenon but is influenced by a complex interplay of hormones and neurotransmitters. Dopamine, for example, has been observed to enhance sexual drive and orgasmic quality, likely by increasing oxytocin release, which plays a role in sexual arousal and orgasm[4]. Medications, such as Cialis and Viagra, can enhance nitrous oxide in the blood, which can make for a more intense orgasm. Understanding the role of these chemicals can lead to targeted treatments that could improve orgasmic response.

---

4   https://www.ncbi.nlm.nih.gov/pmc/articles/PMC11035123/

Difficulty orgasming is called anorgasmia. In some cases, medical treatments may be necessary to address orgasmic difficulties. For instance, a drug called cabergoline has shown promise in treating orgasm problems in men by potentially enhancing dopamine's effect on sexual function.[5]

Shockwave therapy has been shown to improve erections by enhancing blood flow and stimulating the nerves responsible for feeling sexual pleasure. Research is still ongoing on how effective Shockwave Therapy can be for treating anorgasmia, however many of my patients who use Shockwave for ED have reported increased sensation in their penis. To find out more about being a part of our observational studies on Shockwave Therapy, visit https://comprehensive-urology. com/clinical-trials/.

4.   Erectile Dysfunction (ED)

Now that we have an understanding of how healthy erections happen, let's explore the reasons that your erections might not be as full and consistent as they once were. The United States has the highest rate of ED when compared to other developed nations, affecting an estimated 30 million American men[6].

---

5   https://www.health.harvard.edu/
     blog/a-new-option-for-orgasm-problems-in-men-201205294804
6   https://www.niddk.nih.gov/health-information/urologic-diseases/
     erectile-dysfunction/definition-facts

As illustrated in the graph below, age is a major risk factor for ED. However, the US has a higher ED rate when compared to Australia and European nations. The decline of sexual function is observed in the majority of the US male population between their 40s and 80s, and is connected to an unhealthy lifestyle that leads to cardiovascular disease, obesity, and diabetes. However, the general public isn't aware of the recent advances in sexual medicine, which makes ED more treatable than in the past. There's more than just pills to help you recover your sexual ability.

Let's look at the data to see how many men experience ED for each age group.

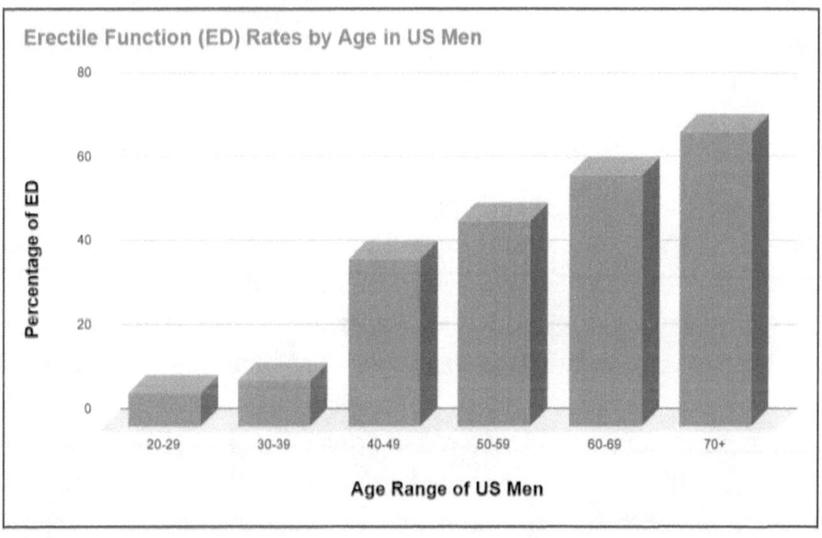

Diagram 2: *Erectile Dysfunction Rates by Age in US Men Bar Graph*

*Chart was compiled from multiple sources specific to each age group. Research on ED rates is ongoing[7] [8] [9].

---

7   https://www.ncbi.nlm.nih.gov/pmc/articles/PMC5313296/
8   https://www.ncbi.nlm.nih.gov/pmc/articles/PMC5313305/
9   https://www.amjmed.com/article/S0002-9343(06)00689-9/pdf

EARLY AGE ED IN YOUR 20S & 30S

ED can happen to any adult man, though it's more prevalent in older men. That being said, there is a rise of ED in men in their 20s and 30s. About 8% of American men in their 20s and 11% of men in their 30s are experiencing some degree of ED.

I've observed among my younger patients that these gentlemen in their twenties and thirties show up because they've noticed that their erections are slowly getting weaker. The softening of erections and your erections lasting a shorter period of time are often the first signs that some part of your body needs to be checked. Intervening early means that we have more tools at our disposal to address the issue. Getting help early produces outcomes and greater longevity for your sex life. If you notice a change, then a change is happening. Ask for help.

After doing a comprehensive approach and identifying where the root causes for these young men, one of the main modalities that we've used has been Shockwave Therapy. Young men in their 20s-30s are typically very sexually active, however when they experience the early stages of ED, they stop dating because of a lack of confidence. This is a prime time in a man's life to learn how to develop intimacy and to potentially establish a meaningful relationship. Many young patients with soft or infrequent erections have shared with me that they go out on dates, but the relationship doesn't advance very far in terms of intimacy sexually because they don't want to fail during sex. So they tend to avoid opportunities for greater physical intimacy and enter into the friend zone. Without a deepening of intimacy, ultimately these relationships break up because the partner doesn't feel like they are wanted.

So returning sexual function at all ages, especially when young men are exploring the possibility of a long-term relationship, is interlinked with their ability to experience intimacy that can lead to greater emotional support.

50% OF MEN BY AGE 50 HAVE ED

We see gentlemen in their forties and fifties who have been in relationships for a long period of time. Up to about 50% of men by the age of 50 will have some degree of erectile dysfunction. So, half of the middle-aged men out there will have doubts about their ability to perform sexually in the way that they desire. Men in long-term relationships who don't feel confident when being sexual start to pull back from intimate moments in that relationship. The partner then feels rejected that their sexual advances aren't supported or well-received. The partner often begins to have doubts about their desirability. This can lead to insecurity that perhaps their male partner wants a younger woman. This particular downward emotional spiral isn't actually caused by the man's desire to have sex with other people or even that he is losing attraction for his mate. He's feeling insecure about his ability to perform sexually, and is embarrassed to talk about it directly because he's been conditioned to believe that he's less of a man for having ED. Nothing could be further from the truth, as ED is a sign that your body needs help. Denying yourself medical care only makes the situation worse physically as well as increases the emotional angst in the relationship.

My male patients in this situation tell me, "Look, I love my partner. We're in love. We've been together for so long, and overall our partnership is fantastic. The problem is that we're not being sexually active." As a urologist, I understand that I might be the only person this man is going to share their secret struggle. So I make sure to have a thorough conversation about it by asking more specific questions about their sexual difficulties. Nine times out of 10, the patient will eventually share, "I'm not feeling sexually confident because my erections aren't so good." Once they admit their struggle with ED, the door is open to address it effectively.

The partner also suffers from their man's ED, more so if they don't know that it's happening. From the partner's perspective, they aren't necessarily thinking that he's struggling with his erections. They're thinking, "he's not being sexual. Does he still love me? Doesn't he care about me? Maybe I'm not attractive anymore, or he's attracted to somebody else." These doubtful questions swirl inside the partner's head incessantly, making them feel lonely and anxious.

In reality, these men aren't falling out of love with their partners, nor do they find them unattractive. They just don't want to fail sexually because they have been conditioned to believe that not being able to deliver an erection during intercourse makes them less of a man.

If they don't ask for professional help for their ED, many men will find subconscious excuses not to engage with their partner. This leaves the partner feeling emotionally rejected and unwanted, even though that is not how the man truly feels about them. Nor did he intentionally want to make them feel dejected. It's just that he's enthralled in a silent struggle and doesn't want you to see him as less of a man.

Once the ED treatments begin to take effect, those doubtful questions go away once they start having sex again. The man's confidence comes back, and they're able to be intimate again and again. The beauty is that recovering their confidence translates into an improved relationship at home. The home situation improved dramatically. The partner feels desired (and blissfully fatigued). And my patients feel in touch with their inner studs.

It's great to see how directly talking about ED can lead to effective treatment. The increase in confidence creates a ripple effect in so many different aspects of a man's life.

SEX IN YOUR 60S AND 70S

Let's talk about our older gentlemen in their sixties and seventies. About 60% of men experience ED in their 60s, and about 70% of men in their 70s have ED. Many of our patients who are 60 or 70 years of age, or even older, just assume that they've lost their ability to have normal sexual function. They resign themselves to thinking this is part of normal aging. This outdated mentality made more sense in their parents' and grandparents' generations, when there were literally no effective medical treatments available for ED. But why party like it's 1899? We have modern medical interventions that are highly effective, so why not take advantage of them?

A popular component to treating my ED patients in their 60s and 70s are medications like Cialis and Viagra. A common concern among my patient's partners is that they're afraid that these medications like Cialis and Viagra can put them at risk of having a heart attack or a stroke. But, in fact, the opposite is true. Both Viagra and Cialis were originally developed to lower blood pressure by relaxing the veins. This means that the heart has less pressure on it and that these medications are cardio-protective. They actually reduce the risk of heart attack and stroke. Educating the partner about their concerns can open more treatment options and increase support for the patient as they undergo ED treatment.

SEX IN YOUR 80S

While many erroneously believe that senior people do not have an active sex life, the steepest rise in sexually transmitted infections (STIs) in the US has been in people 60 years of age and older. STIs are rising in nursing homes, prompting medical staff to make condoms more available to residents[10].

This is all to say that not only is it possible to have a healthy sex life in your 80s, but the prevalence of sex in our later years is increasing, especially amongst those who are utilizing the latest therapies in sexual medicine.

People are living longer thanks to advances in modern medicine as a whole. We also have more treatments for sexual health than ever before. My goal as a urologist is to extend the youthful longevity of my patients well into their elder years. This includes my patients in their 80s. I always seek to defy the rising bar chart that shows ED rates going up with each additional decade of age. I want my patients to be the ones who aren't a part of the majority who are struggling to maintain erections. Rather, I want my patients to be the special few who live with optimized sexual performance.

ED interventions for men in their 80s often involve a combination of therapies, including medications and Shockwave Therapy. But we also have surgical options available as well as Platelet-Rich Plasma (PRP) penile injections that are showing great promise. More on these treatments shortly.

---

10   https://www.ncbi.nlm.nih.gov/pmc/articles/PMC7177870/

HOPE FOR ED

Since men tend to suffer in silence when it comes to ED, they typically come to me after they've had erectile dysfunction for 5 or 10 years. This is self neglect which can limit our treatment options and outcomes. So don't wait to get checked out by your urologist or PCP. The sooner you come to us, the more we can help you, and the longer your sexual function will last. Your sexual enjoyment and vitality are important.

In the cases of patients who've had ED for a few to several years, it could have been an easy fix five or 10 years ago. But by the time they see me, they've progressively taken more and more medications to the point that they're not responsive anymore. These men have essentially lost all hope.

When we talk to them about all the different treatments that we can offer, from anti-aging process hormonal optimization to circulatory optimization, it sparks their hope that it's not too late to get treated. Ever since I started incorporating low-intensity Shockwave Therapy in combination with other treatments, my patients are hopeful that they can revive their sex life. Gentlemen would need between six sessions for moderate ED, up to 12 sessions if they have very severe erectile dysfunction. The treatments can be done every few weeks until complete, and normally patients return once every 6–12 months to maintain results.

The best part of non-invasive Shockwave Therapy is there's absolutely zero downtime. You can go home and have same-day sex. So many of those men who had lost hope have become sexually active again. 80% of my patients respond to the treatment, providing them with solid erections with an increase in girth and their length because blood flow is drastically improved. They're able to achieve erections naturally. No pills. No surgery.

By intervening early with ED, we're able to reverse that aging process. Many men are capable of getting off medications before they become resistant to their effects. We're able to improve the overall circulatory health, and with Shockwave Therapy, a much better state of penal circulation locally. I love to see the confidence come back again in the eyes of my patients after they see the results a comprehensive treatment of ED can bring. We'll talk about Shockwave Therapy in detail later in the book.

Just remember that there is hope to recover your sexual function. The sooner you ask for help, the better the results. If you have a more severe case that has lasted for years, we can use a combination of therapies to address all the contributing factors to your ED.

Youth is not that far away.

So regardless of a man's age, we can restore youthful sexual function instead of waiting for a slow decline of our sexual ability. We can help your body improve naturally using a combination of customized treatment options to ensure satisfying sex at almost any age.

WHY NATURAL ERECTIONS ARE SUPERIOR TO ASSISTED ERECTIONS

A natural erection is always best. Why?

Natural erections are as nature intended. They arrive on time and do so reliably when a man is in a good state of health. Most importantly, natural erections are powered by your own hormone-infused blood flow. The longer you can produce erections naturally, the longer your active sex life will last. I save the more potent treatments, such as surgical penile implants, for men who have had significant decline of their erectile function and have exhausted all the other possibilities.

The ultimate goal should be not only to help a gentleman have excellent erections but to be able to help them do so naturally with less reliance on medications with less reliance on surgical intervention. This is now possible by using a multimodal approach that checks all the boxes, including the aforementioned optimization of testosterone level, overall circulatory health, and improving local circulation to the penis using Shockwave Therapy. Modern sexual medicine is all about optimizing sexual health as naturally as possible by using a comprehensive, multimodal approach. If we're able to help your body heal itself and reverse its aging process, it's better for you as it minimizes side effects and extends the shelf life of your body parts. Each patient is unique, so putting together a personalized health plan will always work best.

Let's talk about the factors that contribute to ED.

PSYCHOLOGICAL IMPACT ON ED

In the same way that the arousal process begins with psychological and sensory stimulation, mental distress can derail that process. Mental anguish and unexpressed emotions can put us in an agitated state that interrupts the brain's ability to send signals to the body when it's time to engage. We need to relax to fully arrive at the moment with a sufficient erection.

Work stress is a leading cause of mental strain that can interrupt intercourse. Having too much on your mind and not being able to switch your brain off will prevent you from feeling the sensations in your body. Unwinding before intercourse in the form of meditation, yoga, or even working out with your partner can loosen you up.

But sometimes the level of mental training is too great to discharge with daily practice. This is where therapy can really shine because you can unburden your stresses and clear your mind of your worries so that when you come home, you're ready to enjoy sex.

As I mentioned earlier, performance anxiety can make a man worry about whether he will satisfy his partner. This mental stress can prevent an erection from happening because you're putting too much pressure on yourself at the moment. Try a five-minute breathing exercise before you go to bed. Inhale for a count of seven seconds, hold your breath for a count of eight seconds, then exhale for a count of four seconds. This naturally switches the brain from the fight-or-flight response to the parasympathetic mode of the nervous system. By releasing your mind, the nerves tell the body that it's time to relax. Erections are more likely to happen in this calm state of mind.

One of the biggest emotional blocks towards achieving satisfying erections is shame. Shame can interrupt your ability to engage sexually and create distance in your relationships. Some people feel guilty or ashamed about being sexual or about having naughty fantasies. Having fantasies and sexual curiosities is a normal part of being human. This shame can come from religious beliefs or their prior sexual history, including past abuse or feelings of rejection from past relationships. Talking about the shame with a trusted supporter or practitioner begins to move the shame out of your mind.

Not all erectile dysfunction stems from a physical problem. There are often external stressors preventing our bodies from cooperating in sexual situations. I had a male patient struggling to get erections with his wife. Upon exploring potential causes, he admitted he wasn't feeling attracted to his wife. The stress of a potentially failing marriage weighed so heavily on him that it was materializing physically. I recommended him to a therapist, and after doing the inner work, he found he was dealing with a combination of past trauma and increased life stressors. His therapist worked with him to manage his stress and reduce his anxiety. Identifying the root of the problem beyond the mere physical condition is ultimately what brought him a solution. He wrote to me later saying this emotional work is what healed his relationship with his wife and rejuvenated their physical intimacy.

Psychological factors, such as anxiety and stress, can profoundly affect a man's ability to reach orgasm. Men who have difficulty reaching ejaculation/orgasm often cite stress as a putative reason for their problem[11]. It's essential to clear the mental slate, to clear your mind before engaging in sex. Exercise, yoga, and meditation can all help clear the mental slate.

PENILE CIRCULATION – THE PENIS IS A VASCULAR ORGAN

There's a good reason that you don't walk around with a full erection all day. It would get in the way of your daily life. And having an erection for more than four hours isn't healthy, as it can starve the cells of your penis from receiving oxygen brought by fresh blood. To have an erection, your penis must be filled with blood. All the vascular tissue, including blood vessels, flood with blood so that the penis becomes engorged. So if there is an issue with the blood vessels or problems with blood flow in your circulatory system, you will have struggles achieving and maintaining a satisfying erection. Many patients have

---

11   https://www.ncbi.nlm.nih.gov/pmc/articles/PMC10318491/

issues with their cardiovascular health, which can eventually impact the blood flow to your penis, resulting in ED.

So when we're able to help our patients with a comprehensive approach, one of the modalities that we use most frequently is low-intensity Shockwave Therapy. With Shockwave Therapy, we're able to naturally re-institute their normal circulatory function.

How does that work? We use a device that's placed on the penis externally, an extremely comfortable procedure, that takes about 20 to 30 minutes. It's literally that easy. After six sessions, a considerable number of our patients will come back and say, "You know what? My erections are great. I'm able to get morning erections again. I'm able to last as long as I want. I'm confident." What happens is that the relationships at home transform. Why? Because they're confident. Again, they know that they can sexually perform, they know that they can be what they want to be in the bedroom.

DRUGS

Many men who use recreational drugs or too many prescription painkillers complain of difficulty achieving strong erections. It's difficult to arrive with a lasting erection when someone is drunk or under the influence of stronger drugs, like cocaine and MDMA.

MDMA, also known as Ecstasy or Molly, is a synthetic drug that raises many neurotransmitters (brain hormones) that increase empathy and emotional expression and can give a short state of euphoria. However, as it temporarily raises neurotransmitters such as dopamine (the reward hormone), serotonin (the happiness hormone), and norepinephrine (the alert hormone that turns on the lights in your brain), it can lead to a hard crash six hours later. This withdrawal can disrupt sleep and the ability to have erections as the body scrambles to rebalance its neurotransmitters. Just like SSRIs, including Prozac and Zoloft, MDMA raises your serotonin levels and can have the side effect of crippling your erections.

Continued drug and alcohol abuse can degrade your brain's ability to send the necessary signals to form an erection. Unhealthy habits can harm your cardiovascular system responsible for managing the blood flow that creates your erection and can even disrupt your positive mindset necessary to reach that calm mental state to produce a reliable erection.

Healthy studs have healthy erections!

PHYSICAL EXERCISE

Physical health and fitness can play a significant role in sexual performance. Cardiovascular exercise, in particular, can improve blood flow and stamina, both of which are important for sexual health and the ability to have stronger orgasms.

Getting a full work-up with your cardiologist is essential to ensuring optimal sexual performance. A healthy heart and lungs lead to a healthy stud.

Pelvic Floor Exercises: Strengthening the Foundation of Your Genitals

The pelvic floor is a group of muscles that play a vital role in supporting the organs, controlling bladder and bowel function, and even enhancing sexual function. Pelvic floor exercises, also known as Kegel exercises, are a simple yet effective way to strengthen these important muscles and improve overall pelvic health.

Pelvic floor exercises involve the voluntary contraction and relaxation of the muscles that make up the pelvic floor. As described by the Mayo Clinic, "Kegel exercises can strengthen the pelvic floor muscles, which support the bladder and bowel and affect sexual function." By engaging and strengthening these muscles, individuals can experience a range of proven benefits.

One of the primary benefits of pelvic floor exercises is improved bladder control. As noted by the Cleveland Clinic, "Kegel exercises can give you better control over your bladder and bowels and prevent your pelvic muscles from getting weak." This can be particularly helpful for individuals experiencing urinary incontinence or pelvic organ prolapse.

In addition to bladder control, pelvic floor exercises have also been shown to enhance sexual function. Pelvic floor exercises have also been associated with reduced pelvic pain, improved core stability, and even enhanced enjoyment during sexual intercourse[12].

MAIN ERECTILE DYSFUNCTION CAUSES:

1. ED Circulatory Issues:
    Erectile dysfunction ensues because the blood flow to the penis is limited. The penis is a very vascular organ. So if a gentleman cannot achieve or maintain erections to their satisfaction, that's a hallmark that the blood flow to the penis is now diminished and just not satisfactory anymore. Why does that happen? Suppose somebody has a circulatory issue or is at risk for circulatory issues such as diabetes, high cholesterol level, hypertension, just to name a few. In that case, they're going to be at risk not just as a whole organ system to their heart, to their kidneys, to their brain, but

---

12   https://www.mayoclinic.org/healthy-lifestyle/mens-health/in-depth/
      kegel-exercises-for-men/art-20045074

also to their penis, which means that the blood flow to the penis can and is compromised if they're noticing that the erections are not particularly strong. Two, some of the nerve endings that are important to allow the blood flow to actually circulate properly can also be affected, particularly in gentlemen who have diabetes.

2. Hormone Stability (Low T and Low Thyroid):
    Hormonal instability, including various forms of testosterone and thyroid hormones, can disrupt our ability to engage in sex and can cause changes to our metabolism, resulting in muscle loss and fat gain. So if a gentleman has, for example, low testosterone level or if their thyroid functions are off, they can experience inadequate erections.

3. Psycho-social Well-being:
    To correctly diagnose and properly implement a treatment plan for a patient, we have to take a look at a patient comprehensively. How are they doing psychosocially? What is their activity level like? What are the other co-founding variables within their health?

By understanding the causes of ED, we can encourage lifestyle changes and the use of minimally invasive therapies to arrive at natural erections. We can also use more potent therapies to recover sexual function when the less invasive interventions aren't working well enough.

ERECTILE DYSFUNCTION TREATMENTS

Now that we've covered the most common psychological and overall physical health issues that contribute to ED, let's get into the treatment options.

Our clinic is a popular choice for second and even third opinions for patients seeking help with erectile dysfunction. The knee-jerk response of most physicians is just to prescribe Viagra or Cialis without doing a full evaluation to see what is the core issue behind the ED. We approach things from a completely different mindset as we seek to optimize the patient's natural ability to have satisfying erections.

Proper treatment starts with a full assessment of what's causing the dysfunction.

Our comprehensive approach begins by tracking all the physiological changes that are happening in a gentleman's body. Once we can track the imbalances and dysfunctions, the question becomes how do we start to reverse and delay them? I'm constantly asking myself, "what can we do, from an anti-aging perspective, to help a man naturally have much better erections with less reliance on medications?"

I'll give you a peek inside my mind as I assess a new patient who is suffering from ED:

Hormonal Status: What's happening with my patient's endocrine system? How are their testosterone levels, including their free T and total T. Is their metabolism slowing down? Let's check their thyroid hormone.

Circulatory Health: How are the heart and lungs doing? How's the blood flow to their penis?

Nerve Health: Are the nerves responding properly? Are they being damaged by sluggish blood circulation? Are they losing sensitivity which would stop them from responding to physical stimulation? Could Shockwave Therapy help?

Stress Levels: Is my patient under pressure at work? Are there relationship conflicts or signs of performance anxiety that might be helped with therapy?

Physical Damage: Is my patient's penis bent (Peyronie's disease) which could be a sign of physical trauma that is causing ED?

Our goal has to be to reverse imbalances and degradation of a healthy system as much as possible. So we take a look at their baseline function, we take a look at their risk factors, we take a look at their quality of life in terms of behaviors and how active they are in order to get to our patients as an individual. Every case is different. Every patient can benefit from a comprehensive assessment of their health status.

One of the other key elements that we start to take a look at is to see if they are a candidate for low-intensity Shockwave Therapy (a.k.a. PulseWave Therapy). Using an apparatus that emits soundwaves to stimulate new blood vessel growth (angiogenesis) and positively stimulate the nerves for a more responsive penis.

A typical course of Shockwave Therapy treatment includes one to two times a week for six sessions. Each session takes about 20 to 30 minutes and is essentially painless. After the outpatient treatment, people get up, go home, and are able to have same-day sex with no downtime. I love hearing back the feedback of our patients when they are once again having the best sex of their lives. Many of them come into the office just to give us a big hug to thank us for helping them with such a sensitive issue. Some kind things our patients have shared are:

> *You gave me back my sexual life.*
> *You've given my confidence back to me.*
> *I am so happy now that I'm dating again.*

I'm much more active, and I'm so much better with my partner.

As a physician, these "thank yous" mean the world to me. I love helping my patients find their youth again and the confidence to engage in sex naturally without being dependent on pills or injections. That's the difference that comprehensive care makes.

5.   ED Treatments

Now let's delve into the various treatments that we use on a daily basis for our ED patients at Comprehensive Urology in Los Angeles.

RIDING THE WAVES OF SHOCKWAVE THERAPY

Low-Intensity Shockwave Therapy for ED, (a.k.a. Pulse Wave Therapy) is an ingenious way to naturally optimize erections. If a body part is repeatedly stimulated with Shockwave Therapy, the body creates new blood vessels in that area. Imagine, if you clap your hands repeatedly. Over time, the palm of your hand turns red. Why does that happen?

The skin flushes red because it's responding to this repeated stimulation by increasing the blood flow to the area. This increased blood flow results in your palm becoming red. If this is repeated over time, not only does your body increase blood flow to the area, it also starts to create new blood flow channels to the area as well. We can therefore use this concept to increase the blood flow to the penis. We can send repeated pulsewaves (4,500-5,000 small impulses) to the penis over a 15-minute period.

With repeated stimulations, your body is triggered to increase the blood flow to the penis as well as create new blood flow channels to it. Both result in increased blood flow and blood carrying capacity resulting in improved erections. PulseWave Therapy is extremely well tolerated and has no downtime. In repeated double-blind scientific studies, the results demonstrate

that approximately 80% of men undergoing PulseWave Therapy get significant improvement in their erections[13]. Even men without erectile dysfunction can gain benefit from it by being able to have firmer erections. Some men who undergo PulseWave Therapy also describe that their penis appears larger in length or girth, and that they are able to last longer when having sex.

Many men prefer to improve their erections naturally and not to be dependent on lifelong medications. PulseWave Therapy can be a great way to naturally improve erections without dependence on medications. Other men who are using medications, and want to improve their erections without taking additional medications can also benefit from PulseWave Therapy. Many of them are able to get better erections with a combination of medications and pulse wave therapy.

Other men, who have such severe erectile dysfunction that they don't respond to medications, can use pulse wave therapy to improve their penile blood flow to the point that they can become responsive to medications like Viagra or Cialis. Lastly, many men use pulse wave therapy as a preventative measure, including men who are going to undergo prostate surgery and want to minimize their risk of developing erectile dysfunction with surgery.

---

13   https://journals.sagepub.com/doi/10.1177/15579883221087532

Shockwave therapy is really an amazing bit of technology. Let's talk about how this was started. Shockwave therapy was first tried out on people who had inflammation or fasciitis in the soft tissue of their body. Say that their shoulder muscle was inflamed from an injury. That patient would receive small pulses of low-intensity shockwaves throughout that tissue using a pulsewave device. They discovered that the shockwaves stimulated blood flow and ultimately increased vascular growth of new blood vessels into that particular tissue.

The body responds by improving the blood flow to that area in response to the sound waves stimulating it by building new blood vessels. These new blood flow channels allow the inflammation to flow out of the inflamed area and restore blood flow.

So some genius said, "If I apply this Shockwave Therapy to the penis, what will happen to this vascular organ that is full of blood vessels?"

A new therapy for penile rejuvenation was born, giving hope to millions of men experiencing ED.

By repeatedly sending these painless sound waves into the penis, you tell the body, "I need more blood flow here." The result is improved blood flow to the penis and erections start to naturally enhance. Just a few treatments are able to build new blood vessels and new pathways for blood to flow. This is why the positive effects last long-term after just a few treatments, because you're not going to lose new blood vessels overnight. More blood flow means faster healing and growth of new cells in your penis.

Remember that the penis itself is just a vascular organ with multiple different vessels inside. So new growth of blood vessels will have a much more dramatic effect than applying it to cartilage that has very little blood flow. So if a man's erectile function is going down, that's a sign that the blood flow to the penis is being compromised. In the past, the only things we could potentially do was to give somebody Viagra or Cialis, but then they would become dependent on these medications for increased blood flow.

The natural blood flow to a man's penis starts to diminish with age, which means that a man would then need higher and higher and higher doses of these medications until they just stop responding because they reached the maximum benefit from the pills. Once this happens, we need to go to secondary or even third-line therapies. What has been missing is our ability to be able to naturally reverse that aging cycle and improve the overall circulation within the penis itself. We just didn't have the technology until the past few years. Now that we have Shockwave Therapy, the ED recovery process has become much simpler by focusing on the body's ability to build new blood vessels rather than opening up the pre-existing ones with Viagra or Cialis.

The treatment is completely painless. The whole procedure takes about 15 to 20 minutes to complete using a handheld device that sends painless sound waves into the penis.

Some feedback I often get from my patients after trying Shockwave Therapy for the first time:

> *I'm waking up with morning erections again.*
> *I'm getting much harder erections.*
> *I don't need to take my medications anymore.*
> *I feel extremely confident now with my sexual ability*

We even have patients tell us that their penis is longer and wider than they remember. This is perhaps because the new blood vessels are filling their penis to the maximum, whereas before they were missing out on full erections because of decreased blood flow. Once you reestablish that blood flow, the erection enhancement happens naturally. With greater blood flow, the body is more capable of healing itself.

Every time I can get a patient off of medications for assisted erections, I celebrate because that patient is optimizing their sexual health. It means that I did my job to the fullest as their doctor.

SHOCKWAVE THERAPY RECOVERY TIME

Shockwave therapy is painless and patients go home the same day. There's no downtime and men are free to have same-day sex on the day of the treatment. After the treatment, they get up, go home, and are able to be sexually active. Many men notice a tingling sensation after the treatment, but no other side effects have been found in studies.

How long does it take to see results with Shockwave Therapy?

The maximum results after the initial treatment arrive about 12 weeks later. Why? Because Shockwave Therapy itself is actually stimulating blood flow creation within the penis, which requires new capillaries (the smallest blood vessels) to be created. This takes a couple of months for the body to do. And when we do that, we're stimulating the body to start this process. With the new blood vessels, we reach a new steady state of the blood flow to the penis.

The beauty of Shockwave Therapy's results is that this will continue for a longer period of time after treatments because the new blood vessels continue to do their job for the next couple of years. The majority of our patients, even two years out, are still noticing the positive benefits of the treatment. For many men, they decide that they want to go on a maintenance program where they come in every six months to preserve the benefits for years to come. Shockwave therapy has been a game changer for many of my patients. Confidence comes back, spontaneity in their sex life revives back, and they're able to function like they are 10 or 15 years younger.

Key Takeaways of Shockwave Therapy

1. Extremely easy to do: takes about 20 to 30 minutes. You feel just about nothing. You get up, you go home, you're back to your normal life.
2. Highly effective: approximately 80% of the men that we use this for say, "I'm getting up with the morning erection, now my erections are harder. I'm able to maintain them." Its effects are long-lasting, an initial series of treatments can last a few years. Most men only need a tune-up treatment every six months to maintain results for years to come.
3. Increased girth and length: for many men, their girth and length are better.
4. Boosts your confidence: it is incredibly important for men to have normal sexual functions. It improves, it helps improve their confidence level on so many different levels.
5. Fast recovery, same-day sex: after you get the treatment done, literally minutes later you're back to your normal self. You want to get busy, get busy.

PENILE INJECTIONS FOR ED

In the past, when patients failed using oral medications like Viagra and Cialis, the next level of medications for assisted erections were injectables. These early penile injections are still used today by urologists to check the functionality of the penis in its erect state. This physical exam entails a small injection into the penis which facilitates an assisted erection without arousal nor physical stimulation. This helps your physician to see if you're having blood flow issues or if the cause behind your ED might be caused by another condition.

Oral medications stimulate the nerves to release more nitric oxide, which in turn causes the penile blood vessels to open up and allow more blood into the penis. If these medications don't work, then we can bypass the nerves and directly stimulate the penile vessels to open up. We do this by injecting the penis with three medications (TriMix) that in concert directly cause the penile vessels to open up. At first thought, imagining that someone is going to inject the penis sounds horrifying. But in reality, we use a tiny needle and the injection isn't more than just a tiny sting. The whole process takes about five seconds. The result for most men is getting a solid erection within 15 minutes from the time of the injection. About 10% of men complain of penile aches after an injection. For these men, we change the formulation of the three medications and most will be comfortable with the new formulations.

These injectable medications are often a combination of two or more medications to maximize the resulting erection. The most commonly used injectable medication is TriMix. Anyone who finds that TriMix is ineffective may be prescribed QuadMix.

Assisted Erection Injections Include:

- BiMix (papaverine and phentolamine)
- TriMix (papaverine, phentolamine, and prostaglandin E1)
- QuadMix (TriMix and atropine)

I reserve these medications as a last resort because it's always preferable to restore the natural ability to have health erections. In the same way that patients can become dependent on oral medications such as Viagra and Cialis, your body can become reliant on injections for assisted erections.

Fortunately, sexual medicine has seen some promising initial results with the rise of reparative penile injections. Though these new types of injections are also injected into the penis using a small syringe, what is happening inside the penis is drastically different.

New Types of Penis Injections

Remember the name of the game to get a good erection is to get improved blood flow to the penis. So, if oral medications (like Viagra, Cialis, Levitra, Stendra) are not effective enough and despite Shockwave Therapy, you're not getting satisfactory, hard erections, then we can consider reparative penile injections.

Reparative penis injections don't directly force your penis into an erect state using medications as seen in TriMix-like medications. Instead, they trigger an immune response and stimulate the growth of new cells inside the penis itself. Over time, many men have found that they begin recovering their natural ability to have satisfying erections, in some cases even going off medications for ED.

Penile injections have emerged as a potential treatment option for men suffering from ED. Two specific types of penile injections that have been explored for this purpose are Platelet-Rich Plasma (PRP) injections and Botox (botulinum toxin) injections.

Platelet-Rich Plasma (PRP) injections involve extracting a patient's own blood, separating out the platelet-rich component, and then re-injecting it into the penis. The goal is to stimulate tissue regeneration and improve blood flow, which can help restore erectile function. A study published in Urology found that "PRP injection therapy improved erectile function in men with mild to moderate ED." The researchers concluded that PRP penile injections may be a "safe and effective minimally invasive option" for treating certain cases of ED. Let's explore each type of penile injection in detail.

BOTOX PENILE INJECTIONS FOR ERECTILE DYSFUNCTION

Botox, the brand name for the neurotoxin botulinum toxin, has also been explored as a potential treatment for erectile dysfunction. When injected into the penis, Botox is thought to relax the smooth muscle tissue, improving blood flow and facilitating erections. A retrospective case series published in MDPI found that "intracavernosal injections of botulinum toxin A (BTX/A ic) may be effective for difficult-to-treat erectile dysfunction (ED)." Additionally, a report from i-Base noted that Botox penile injections "improved blood flow and other outcomes in men with moderate to severe erectile dysfunction."

Botox Efficacy

Let's talk about Botox for penis injections. Yes, the same Botox that is used to decrease wrinkles in your face and increase the size of your lips can also potentially help your penis.

Our traditional treatments, such as oral medications, vacuum devices, and surgical procedures, may not always be effective or suitable for all patients. In recent years, Botox (botulinum toxin) injections into the penis have emerged as a way to stimulate the body's ability to repair itself.

When injected into the penis, Botox is thought to relax the smooth muscle of the corpus cavernosum, that spongy tissue inside the penis that's responsible for trapping blood and maintaining an erection. By relaxing this muscle, Botox may improve blood flow and facilitate better erectile function.

Several studies have explored the use of Botox penile injections for the treatment of ED. A retrospective case series published in the journal MDPI examined the safety and efficacy of intracavernosal Botox injections in men with difficult-to-treat ED[14]. The researchers found that this approach "may be effective for difficult-to-treat erectile dysfunction (ED)," with improvements in overall erectile function.

Botox injections can be done with a single injection into the side of the penis[15]. Botox will aid in vasodilation, which means it opens up the blood vessels to let more blood come into the penis.[16] These injections have been shown to help approximately 50% of men with ED[17] [18].

While the initial findings are encouraging, it's important to note that the long-term safety and efficacy of Botox penile injections for ED are still being investigated. Comprehensive Urology is currently conducting observational studies with the hope that these case studies will lead to larger clinical trials in the future. Please visit https://comprehensive-urology.com/clinical-trials/ for more information. It's also important to note that the American Urological Association (AUA) has acknowledged the potential of this approach but has also emphasized the need for more robust clinical trials to fully understand

---

14   https://www.mdpi.com/2072-6651/15/6/382
15   El-Shaer, W. et al. (2021) 'Intracavernous injection of botox® (50 and 100 units) for treatment of vasculogenic erectile dysfunction: Randomized controlled trial', Andrology, 9(4), pp. 1166–1175. doi:10.1111/andr.13010
16   https://onlinelibrary.wiley.com/doi/full/10.1111/andr.13010
17   Abdelrahman, I.F. et al. (2021) 'Safety and efficacy of botulinum neurotoxin in the treatment of erectile dysfunction refractory to phosphodiesterase inhibitors: Results of a andomized controlled trial', Andrology, 10(2), pp. 254–261. doi:10.1111/andr.13104
18   https://onlinelibrary.wiley.com/doi/full/10.1111/andr.13104

its role in the management of erectile dysfunction. The AUA[19] also recommends first trying non-invasive treatment methods, such as oral medications, before considering minimally invasive penile injections that require a few injections.

Patients considering Botox injections for ED should consult their healthcare providers to discuss the potential benefits, risks, and alternative treatment options. As with any medical procedure, it is crucial to weigh the potential risks and benefits and to make an informed decision based on the individual's specific circumstances and medical history. Our team is available to help you find the next treatment options for your individual case.

PRP PENILE INJECTIONS FOR ERECTILE DYSFUNCTION

PRP stands for platelet-rich plasma. Like many of the ED therapies, including Shockwave Therapy and Botox penile injections, PRP was first used to heal injuries in other parts of the body such as muscles, tendons, ligaments, and cartilage. It harnesses the power of platelets, the blood cells which clot blood when we get a cut that also are responsible for helping to rebuild new cells. Their presence in the body also leads to the release of growth factors that are crucial for building new skin, connective tissue, and blood vessels.

Platelets are a major part of the healing factor in the body, contain nutrients factors and co-factors that stimulate the body to start to heal itself. They work in harmony with other elements in the blood to grow new tissue similarly to stem cells, although stem cells are more dramatic in their impact. When we use that in conjunction with other modalities, such as low-intensity Shockwave Therapy, the

---

19   https://www.auanet.org/guidelines-and-quality/guidelines/
     erectile-dysfunction-(ed)-guideline#x8064

results of PRP penile injections can be even better when it comes to enhancing sexual function.

PRP Penile Injection Steps

PRP is very easy to administer:

1. It requires a simple blood draw into a test tube.
2. The test tube of blood is put in a centrifuge to separate the platelets from the rest of the blood.
3. 15 minutes later, the platelets are pulled into a syringe
4. The penis is numbed with topical lidocaine that takes about 2 minutes to take effect
5. A brief series of injections are made around each side of the penis to even distribute the platelets. This typically entails 2–3 dozen injections, each lasting about 1–2 seconds.
6. The whole procedure from start to finish typically takes less than 30 minutes.

PRP AND SHOCKWAVE THERAPY COMBINED FOR ED AND PEYRONIE'S DISEASE

As men age, the blood carrying capacity diminishes more rapidly after 40. Oral medications used to help with erectile dysfunction are a temporary bandage on a progressively worsening underlying issue. To combat the underlying issue of erectile dysfunction, there needs to be an improved blood supply to the penis: a regeneration of blood vessels. Imagine building a brand-new four-lane highway next to an old, pothole-ridden, traffic-filled highway. To do this, a combination of platelet-rich plasma (PRP) and low-intensity Shockwave Therapy is used. The low-intensity Shockwave Therapy is used to create new blood vessels, and PRP is used to increase vascular growth and repair.

Curvature of the penis, or Peyronie's disease, is more common than you'd think,

though rarely discussed as it often comes with a fair share of embarrassment[20].

Often obtained after a sexual trauma, Peyronie's disease can progress rapidly, leading men to have painful, curved erections that are unable to penetrate[21]. After injury, a hard plaque can form that can result in curvature and penile shortening[22]. When these patients are treated quickly with PRP and low-intensity Shockwave Therapy, the growing plaque can be stopped in its tracks and begin to be reversed[23]. Then, PRP is injected to regenerate and improve healing[24]. The combination maximizes new blood vessel growth, increased blood flow, and deep repair of any physical traumas including flushing out the plaque from Peyronie's Disease[25].

Observed Benefits of PRP + Shockwave Therapy:

- More frequent erections, including in the mornings.
- Stronger, harder erections that are fuller.

20   Shaher, H. et al. (2023) 'Is platelet rich plasma safe and effective in treatment of erectile dysfunction? Randomized controlled study', Urology, 175, pp. 114–119. doi:10.1016/j.urology.2023.01.028.
21   https://www.sciencedirect.com/science/article/abs/pii/S0090429523000742
22   Achraf, C., Abdelghani, P.A. and Jihad, P.E. (2022) 'Platelet-rich plasma in patients affected with Peyronie's disease', Arab Journal of Urology, 21(2), pp. 69–75. doi:10.1080/2090598x.2022.2135284.
23   https://www.ncbi.nlm.nih.gov/pmc/articles/PMC10208162/
24   Geyik, S. (2021) 'Comparison of the efficacy of low-intensity shock wave therapy and its combination with platelet-rich plasma in patients with erectile dysfunction', Andrologia, 53(10). doi:10.1111/and.14197.
25   https://onlinelibrary.wiley.com/doi/10.1111/and.14197

- Increased penis girth and length due to growth factors released by the PRP injections and new blood vessel growth stimulated by Shockwave Therapy.

ERECTILE VACUUM DEVICE (PENIS PUMPS)

One of the non-invasive treatments for ED is the use of a penis pump, also known as a vacuum erection device (VED). This suction device can be used alone for men who aren't taking oral ED medications due to contraindications or side effects. VEDs can also be used as part of a comprehensive treatment plan for ED.

According to the American Urological Association, 75% of men using a penis pump can achieve an erection.[26] The principle behind these devices is simple: they create a vacuum around the penis, which draws blood into the two long cylindrical chambers (corpora cavernosa) inside the penis that fill with blood during an erection. A constriction ring is then applied at the base of the penis to maintain the erection by preventing blood from flowing back out.

A long-term study conducted by the National Institutes of Health[27] validated that vacuum constriction devices (penis pumps) are effective for the treatment of ED and impotence. The study concluded that not only do penis pumps provide a solution for erectile dysfunction on a per-use basis, but they also have the potential to contribute to long-term sexual satisfaction.

Moreover, the accessibility and ease of use of penis pumps make them an attractive option for many men. They do not require medication

---

26 https://www.auanet.org/guidelines-and-quality/guidelines/ erectile-dysfunction-(ed)-guideline
27 https://pubmed.ncbi.nlm.nih.gov/8426404/

or surgery, and they can be used on-demand. This is particularly beneficial for those who may have medical conditions that preclude the use of pharmacological treatments or for those who prefer to avoid surgical interventions.

We often use VEDs in conjunction with other therapies, such as Shockwave Therapy, to maximize the potential for natural erections at Comprehensive Urology in Los Angeles. In my experience, combining two or more modalities enhances the outcomes.

ED MEDICATIONS: VIAGRA, CIALIS, LEVITRA

Traditionally, treatment options for erectile dysfunction have been medications. Viagra (sildenafil) and Cialis (tadalafil) were both originally developed to treat high blood pressure. Then, patients began telling their doctors about how they are having frequent and harder erections since beginning the medication. This makes sense because the penis is filled with blood vessels, so a medication that allows more blood flow could help with ED. What makes Viagra and Cialis unique is that they relax the smallest of blood vessels, called capillaries, to reduce high blood pressure and increase blood flow. The areas of our body that are very rich in capillaries include the brain, the lungs, and the penis.

The medication Levitra (vardenafil) works in a similar way as Viagra and Cialis in that it increases blood flow to the penis. The name brand Levitra has been discontinued by the pharmaceutical company due to supply chain issues, but the generic version Vardenafil is still available. It's considered as safe and effective as Viagra.

Studies have found that both Viagra and Cialis are cardio-protective, meaning in addition to helping with erectile dysfunction, they also protect your heart and lungs by reducing the pressure in the blood vessels. They reduce the strain on your heart. Remember that Viagra and Cialis are not used exclusively for ED, as they are blood pressure medications. Don't be surprised to hear that your grandmother is taking Viagra for her high blood pressure.

HOW DO MEDICATIONS LIKE VIAGRA AND CIALIS WORK?

The way that men get an erection is that the nerves of the penis release a molecule called nitric oxide. Nitric oxide in turn causes the vessels to dilate and to let in more blood resulting in an erection. Then the local cells metabolize (breakdown) the nitric oxide. When the nitric oxide levels lower the vessels stop dilating, the penile blood flow slows down and the erection is lost.

Medications like Viagra, Cialis, Levitra and Stendra are all in a class of medications called PDE5-Inhibitors. These medications block the breakdown of the nitric oxide and cause it to stay active for a longer period of time. The increased levels of nitric oxide stimulate the penile blood vessels to open up more and to let increased blood flow in for a longer time, resulting in improved and more sustained erections.

These medications have been revolutionary, as millions of men who have erectile dysfunction have been able to regain their sex life with these medications.

What is the best way to use these medications? These medications can be divided into 2 categories:

1. Short onset and short duration (Viagra, Levitra, and Stendra): onset 30–60 minutes, with an effect that lasts 4–6 hours

2. Slow onset and long duration (Cialis): takes five hours to kick in, and lasts about 24–26 hours

All of these medications work best if taken on an empty stomach. So it's best to take them an hour before you eat anything, or three hours after you have had a meal. What if you have eaten and need to take a short onset medication like Viagra or Levitra but are planning on engaging in sexual activity prior to waiting a few hours for your food to digest first? In cases of "emergency" you can chew the pill, let it sit in your mouth and under your tongue with a drop of oil for a few minutes, then swallow it with some water. The oil has fat in it, which helps it absorb through the skin of your tongue more effectively. Doing so allows the medication to absorb through the lining of your mouth and not be solely dependent on absorbing it through your stomach. By doing so, you can still get good effects from these medications despite having just eaten. However, beware, the pills when chewed will taste bitter. Also, don't try this method for your first time since it can lead to a head rush or dizzy spell. It's best to do this once you've become accustomed to the medication.

What if you need more spontaneity and don't want to time when you need to take medications?

In this case, you can take a lower daily dose of Cialis. With this approach the medication is in you all of the time, allowing more spontaneity. PulseWave Therapy is another great option to allow for more natural, spontaneous erections without the need for medications.

WHAT ARE THE SIDE EFFECTS OF
THESE MEDICATIONS?

For a full list of potential side effects, it's best to look at each medication's package inserts. The main side effects that can occur are:

1. Headache
2. Flushing
3. Stomach acid reflux
4. Muscle aches (mainly with Cialis)
5. Seeing blue colors when looking into the light

Contraindications:

People who take nitrates (mainly for heart disease) should not use these medications.

What if you don't get an erection even with high doses of these medications? First, make sure you are correctly taking these medications (on an empty stomach and waiting the necessary time for the medications to take effect). If you have done so, then you may have severe erectile dysfunction.

ED Medications + Shockwave Therapy

Vardenafil, Cialis, or Viagra combined with Shockwave Therapy offers even greater benefit to patients with ED. As I mentioned before, Shockwave Therapy stimulates angiogenesis, which is the growth of new blood vessels. Think of these new blood vessels as your penis gaining newer, younger parts in the plumbing. When you have a medication that relaxes the blood vessels and a therapy that stimulates new blood vessel creation, you have the ultimate combination of new blood flow in your erections. Simply put, you have harder, more full erections. I've noticed patients achieving an increase in size of their erections as new tissue grows and the medications make the penis more turgid. I've even had the partners of patients thank me for the treatments because they also received the benefits of improved erections.

DR. MICHEL'S CHECKLIST FOR SEVERE ED TREATMENT:

1. Start Shockwave Therapy to improve your penile blood flow to the point you become responsive to medications. Start with 6 treatments administered over a 2-month period.
2. If you still are not responding to Shockwave Therapy, you can start intracorporeal therapy (TriMex penis injections for assisted erections). We've seen great results and are very well tolerated by most patients.
3. If intracorporeal therapy doesn't work, then consider PRP penile injections or Botox penile injections to stimulate your natural ability to repair and achieve erections. It's also possible to combine medications with reparative penile injections.
4. If all previous treatments have failed, then surgery can be considered, such as the placement of a penile implant or inflatable device.

SURGERY FOR ED: PENILE IMPLANTS

Penile implants, also known as penile prosthesis, are a surgical treatment option for erectile dysfunction (ED) when other treatments have been ineffective. These devices are implanted within the erectile chambers of the penis and can be inflated or bent into position to provide an erection suitable for sexual intercourse.

The benefits of penile implants are significant for those suffering from ED. They offer a permanent solution that can lead to high rates of patient and partner satisfaction. Despite their benefits, penile implants come with risks, as with any surgical procedure. The Mayo Clinic[28] also notes that complications such as infection are possible. In rare cases, implant problems such as mechanical failure can occur, necessitating additional surgery. Another potential risk is that implantation may make natural erections difficult to achieve and could limit other treatment options in the future. This is why surgery is always the last resort as we want to preserve the penis' ability to heal and regenerate new tissue, including additional blood vessels.

Overall, penile prosthesis surgery is a safe and effective treatment for patients with erectile dysfunction, particularly in those who are medically complex. This suggests that while there are risks associated with penile implants, they can be a viable option for a broad range of patients, including those with complex medical backgrounds[29].

I also exhaust all other possibilities before offering my surgical options to many patients. But patients in their 70s or 80s, in particular prostate cancer survivors who have had their prostate removed, may be good candidates for this surgery.

---

28   https://www.mayoclinic.org/tests-procedures/penile-implants/about/
      pac-20384916
29   https://www.ncbi.nlm.nih.gov/pmc/articles/PMC10772644/

PREMATURE EJACULATION:
THE LINK BETWEEN PE AND ED

While Premature Ejaculation (PE) and ED are distinct conditions, they can sometimes co-occur. PE is characterized by ejaculation that happens with minimal sexual stimulation, and it happens before the person wishes. This can lead to decreased satisfaction of their partner, causing distress and frustration about sexual performance. ED, on the other hand, is the inability to achieve or maintain an erection suitable for sexual intercourse.

The psychological impact of ED can sometimes lead to PE because the anxiety and stress from being unable to maintain an erection may lead to a rush to ejaculate. Conversely, the stress of experiencing PE may contribute to ED because of performance anxiety.

The good news is that by resolving the ED, the psychological pressure is reduced and the PE can sometimes resolve. We're currently trying Shockwave Therapy on our PE patients to see if it increases the time to climax and reduces the emotional strain if they also have ED[30].

Other treatment methods for PE include:

1. Traditional treatment with antipsychotic and low-dose pain medication, but these pose a risk of depression and habit formation
2. Numbing spray can be used, but it defeats the purpose of enjoying the pleasure of sex The numbing spray can also make your partner numb, preventing them from climaxing
3. Pelvic floor therapy has been utilized with studies showing it can increase time to ejaculation by two to three times

---

30 https://www.medicalnewstoday.com/articles/
    erectile-dysfunction-and-premature-ejaculation

In our clinic, patients are now treated without lifelong medications by the using three

PRP shots and six sessions of low-intensity Shockwave Therapy[31] in combination. Initial case studies have shown an increased time to ejaculation by two to 3.5 times.

PRP + Shockwave Therapy[32] + pelvic floor rehabilitation exercises are also being used together, which we refer to as the *STUD Protocol* because it maximizes the physical readiness of the patient for intercourse[33].

HOW DO I LAST LONGER WHEN HAVING SEX?

Different people have different set points after which they will reach climax. Typically, the time to orgasm increases with age. However, many men would like to be able to last longer during sexual activity, and there are simple ways that this can be achieved. Most sedatives create a situation where a man lasts longer. That's why we need to talk to some men to see if they've drank a little alcohol, or if they've used any other type of sedative at a mild dose so they were able to last longer. In our practice, we typically use a combination of tramadol as well as a PDE5 inhibitor in combination.

This combination typically works very well for the majority of men. In addition to this, pulse wave

---

31   Geyik, S. (2021) 'Comparison of the efficacy of low-intensity shock wave therapy and its combination with platelet-rich plasma in patients with erectile dysfunction', Andrologia, 53(10). doi:10.1111/and.14197.
32   https://onlinelibrary.wiley.com/doi/10.1111/and.14197
33   Pastore, A.L. et al. (2014) 'Pelvic floor muscle rehabilitation for patients with lifelong premature ejaculation: A novel therapeutic approach', Therapeutic Advances in Urology, 6(3), pp. 83–88. doi:10.1177/1756287214523329.

therapy can also be used that will enhance the effect of these medications even further for most men. When patient's need more support, a low dose of antidepressants, such as Prozac, can be used with good effect for most. Topical anesthetic creams to numb the penis are sometimes used, however, in my opinion, this defeats the purpose of being sexually active as it numbs the nerves that give you pleasure.

6. Peyronie's Disease Treatments

PEYRONIE'S DISEASE

Sometimes called "bent penis disease," Peyronie's Disease is when a man's penis starts to curve unnaturally. Why does it happen? Many Peyronie's Disease patients had a physical sexual trauma that injured the vascular tissue of the penis. This can happen during penetration. For instance, if they miss during a penetration attempt, an injury can form resulting in a plaque that can cause a bend in the penis because that part of the vascular tissue is blocked. Some gentlemen tell us, "Look, I woke up that morning and my penis from that point on was bent." They have no memory of trauma, and the bent penis comes as a surprise. Regardless if you had an injury to the penis recently or not, the bending of the penis due to the formation of plaque needs to be treated to restore the penis' natural state.

HOW DO WE TREAT A BENT PENIS?

Early diagnosis is key to a successful treatment of Peyronie's disease. We want to diagnose it as early as possible because the sooner a gentleman comes in with Peyronie's disease, the easier it is to be able to minimize the progression of bending. Of course, we want to do all we can to straighten the penis as quickly as possible.

Some of the signs that a patient is still within the acute phase is that that area is still tender. That's actually a good sign. It's early: come in and get yourself treated. Does that mean that if it's a little bit more chronic, that it cannot be irreversible? Absolutely not. Obviously, earlier is better than later, but you can still improve. How do we do that? In the past, the only therapies that we had were medications, which are highly ineffective. We had different injections that we put into the penis itself, with significant side effects, or we had surgery.

PEYRONIE'S DISEASE MULTIMODAL TREATMENT:

1. Apply low-intensity Shockwave Therapy to slowly break up that little plaque by sending repeated sound impulses and signs
2. Extenders (traction devices) stretch the penis tissue and the plaque itself to break it up and increase blood flow in the area
3. Viagra or Cialis has been shown in some studies to aid during the acute phase as it flushes out the area and may help move out the plaque

Why use extenders? Imagine if you have a frozen shoulder, you can't move it much, but to be able to again, you should mobilize that shoulder more and more. The range of motion comes back. The same thing is true for a penis that's scarred. We want to open up that scar nonsurgically, and start to stretch it so that the mobility of the penis can improve. This is highly effective and we do it routinely. One of the key elements is this device, low-intensity shockwave treatments. We're able to focus sound waves on the plaque itself. The plaque is the scar tissue. The sound waves repeatedly hit that scar tissue, and they allow it to loosen up. Then, using different forms of penile stretching traction and ultimately plaque mobilization, we can get much more fluidity and mobility in this soft tissue of the penis, allowing the gentleman to have a much straighter erection.

What's important is that for several men with Peyronie's, their condition is preceded by some degree of erectile dysfunction, meaning that the erections weren't perfect even before they had the penal trauma. We find the gentleman has baseline erectile dysfunction, even if it's mild. One of the beauties of low-intensity Shockwave Therapy is that not only does it get rid of the plaque, but at the same time is stimulating increased blood flow to the penis. And by doing so, not only can we get rid of or improve the pliability of the plaque itself and therefore get a better straight erection, but also able to improve a man's circulation naturally and therefore improve their quality of erection, which may have been a significant factor that led to the Peyronie's disease.

Again, the key to effective treatment of Peyronie's disease is early detection and early intervention. If you notice a bend in your penis, this is certainly a sign of Peyronie's disease and should be treated immediately. Contact your urologist as soon as you notice it.

PRP INJECTIONS FOR PEYRONIE'S DISEASE

Platelet-rich plasma (PRP) injections have emerged as a potential treatment for Peyronie's disease. When injected into the area of the fibrous scar tissue inside the penis that causes the curve, it activates a healing process where fresh blood flushes out the plaque build-up.

It also activates a host of hormones, such as IGF-1 (insulin like growth factor) which speeds up the growth of new cells. The concentrated platelets from the PRP injection speeds up tissue repair and regeneration in the area of the traumatized penis.

The rationale behind using PRP injections for Peyronie's disease lies in the natural healing properties of platelets. Platelets are blood components that play a crucial role in wound healing and tissue regeneration. They contain numerous growth factors, including platelet-derived growth factor, transforming growth factor-beta, and vascular endothelial growth factor, which are known to promote cell proliferation and angiogenesis (the formation of new blood vessels).

Clinical evidence supporting the efficacy of PRP injections in Peyronie's disease is still in the early stages, but some studies have shown promising results. For instance, a study published in the journal "Sexual Medicine Reviews" suggests that PRP therapy could be a safe and effective treatment option for Peyronie's disease. This research is still in the early phases and more research is needed to confirm these findings[34].

PRP injections are already being used in clinics, such as Comprehensive Urology in Los Angeles, as part of observational studies for Peyronie's disease. PRP penile injections are minimally invasive and have been shown in a study that the safety profile of PRP injections appears to be acceptable[35]. Another article by the *Urology Times*, reports that PRP injections appear to be a safe and feasible approach to treating patients with Peyronie's disease, particularly those who may not be good candidates for more invasive procedures[36].

---

34   https://www.sciencedirect.com/science/article/abs/pii/S2050052121000032
35   https://pubmed.ncbi.nlm.nih.gov/35778315/
36   https://www.urologytimes.com/view/
      platelet-rich-plasma-appears-safe-feasible-for-peyronie-disease

Research continues for this exciting new therapy that offers the hope of straightening the bent penises of thousands of men.

7. Penis Enlargement

Some of my patients worry about their penis size. This can be a source of self-doubt and creates issues with confidence, both in and out of the bedroom. This comes from a tendency of men to compare themselves to other men, which is a survival habit to make sure that you can survive conflicts. But there is also a competition for mates that is wired into our primal minds. Being able to please a partner means that you are more likely to maintain a relationship with a partner. Knowing that you can satisfy your partner sexually can build emotional security in the relationship.

On a primal level, many men believe that having a big enough penis to fully stimulate and please their partners will make them more desirable. This is why so many men will go through extreme measures if they feel that they can become larger, even resorting to surgeries that have much higher risks than minimally invasive treatments like penile injections and Shockwave Therapy.

The reality is that your genetics are the starting point when determining the size of your phallus. Learn to use it to the best of your ability and choose a compatible partner.

MALE ENHANCEMENT: HOW CAN I MAKE MY PENIS BIGGER?

However, there are things that can be done to optimize natural length and girth in

a resting state beyond your starting point. These modalities include using Shockwave Therapy (a.k.a. PulseWave Therapy) as well as PDE5 inhibitors such as Cialis and Viagra. For men who have suboptimal erections or ED, these modalities are even more effective.

Options to surgically augment testing length and girth are available ranging from injecting a penis with "fillers" to keep the length longer at a baseline. Surgical implants are also available to stretch the penis but can create lopsided results. This means that the shaft may be disproportionately larger than the head of the penis, creating an odd cosmetic outcome where the head looks smaller. We'll discuss these options in detail in a later chapter.

Word to the wise, enhance your function regardless of your size. Many men don't realize that when they have an erection, that they aren't actually achieving their full erection. This means that before you try a risky penile implant surgery, there are many safe ways to ensure that you are maximizing your erections so that you realize your true penis size. Focus on having harder erections, which means you have more blood filling your penis to reach your optimal size.

Having your best erections may also enable you to have better climaxes as more blood flow ensures that all the hormones and biochemicals involved in achieving an orgasm are being delivered at the right time. Reliable and full erections build confidence. Don't worry about your resting length. What matters is achieving your optimal erections so that when you connect with your partner, you can focus on enjoying the beautiful act itself, rather than worrying about your performance.

NON-SURGICAL PENIS ENLARGEMENT

Many of the treatments first used to treat ED had the unexpected side effect of an increase in penis length and girth. This led to studying these modalities as potential non-surgical penis enlargement therapies. What we wanted to know is if the increased size was purely from more blood going into the vascular tissue of the penis, or was the amount of new blood vessel growth and new cell growth enough to make the penis tissue bigger?

Spoiler alert: both are true. The increased circulation to the penis maximizes the erection capability of your current penis. However, repeated treatments of Shockwave Therapy went beyond helping patients with ED get more erections. More treatments stimulate more growth of new blood vessels (angiogenesis). More injections of PRP into the penis stimulated more cell growth from repeated exposure to growth factors that told the body to keep making more penis cells. So the answer depends on how many treatments you do. Patients successfully treated for ED continue treatments both as a preventative and because they like having more girth and length. We now have men who don't have ED coming because they want to maximize the size of their penis. Let's do the deep dive into how these therapies inspire penis growth.

WHAT ARE PENILE INJECTIONS FOR
MALE ENHANCEMENT?

Patients receiving penile injections for ED treatment noticed that their erections seemed larger than they had remembered, Their partners agreed. A few adventurous doctors began observational studies to see if increased growth was possible. I'm one of those doctors.

Part of the reason for the increase in length and girth is that injections stimulate repair in the penile tissues and can increase blood flow during erections. However, other factors lead to unexpected new growth beyond just achieving harder, more full erections. New tissue was being created, stimulating continued growth of the penis. Now, penile injections can also be used to enhance the size of penises.

Penis injections for the purpose of penis enlargement come in 3 main types.

THE 3 MAIN TYPES OF PENIS INJECTIONS
USED FOR ENLARGEMENT INCLUDE:

1. Platelet-Rich Plasma (PRP) Penile Injections: Platelet-Rich Plasma injections used for ED can also be used to stimulate tissue growth and increase penis size.
2. Botox Penile Injections: Botox can be injected into the penis to help treat erectile dysfunction. It also enlarges the penis in both the flaccid state and during an erection. They have grown in popularity for male enhancement treatments.
3. Dermal Filler Injections: These injections use hyaluronic acid-based dermal fillers, similar to those used for facial cosmetic procedures, to increase the girth of the penis.

PRP INJECTIONS AND TRACTION FOR LENGTH

The same combination of treatments for Peyronie's disease to stretch and dissolve the plaque that causes the penis to bend can be used to enhance penis length in healthy penises. As mentioned before, PRP injections drastically increase the number of platelets inside the penis. Normally, platelets are there to clot and repair cuts and bruises to the body. However, with platelets also comes growth factors that stimulate the production of new cells. When a high concentration of platelets are injected into an area of the body, it can speed up repairs to injuries. But even when there isn't extensive injury, the presence of lots of platelets tells the body that this area needs repair and new cell growth. They stimulate new cell growth via growth factors so that your penis can continue to grow.

Penile length has been a topic of conversation and offbeat jokes since humans learned to speak. However taboo it may be to talk about it publicly, your urologist can offer you a safe haven to explore the new options available to you. Now, there is a simple way to not only add length, but also girth to your penis.

Here's the regime we're currently using at Comprehensive Urology for PRP injections:

One PRP injection per month, administered on a monthly basis for 6 months.

In conjunction with these treatments, there is also some homework to do, gentleman. A vacuum device and a counter traction device will be used at home to help stretch the tissue daily. When this is done for six months, we've seen men gain on average 0.8 inches (2 cm) in length and 0.5 inches (1.3 cm) in girth[37]. Most men erroneously believe that they can only grow a little bit longer, but we've seen noticeable increase in girth with both PRP injections and even more so in Botox Injections[38].

BOTOX PENILE INJECTIONS FOR GROWTH

Botox injections work a little differently than PRP injections for growth. Botox is the injection of botulinum toxin, which stimulates an immune response alone with increased blood flow into the penis. Botox gives a fuller look to the penis in a similar way that it pushes out wrinkles in your skin or increases the volume of the lips. The inflammation, when done in the right amount, can be beneficial as it expands the penis in both the resting and erect states. The renewed blood flow not only makes achieving erections easier but also makes for a larger erection[39].

Botulinum toxin, commonly known as Botox, is a neurotoxic protein that has various medical and cosmetic applications. In recent years, Botox has been explored as a treatment for erectile dysfunction (ED) and as a means to enhance penile size. The use of Botox for these purposes is relatively novel, and while some studies suggest potential benefits, it is important to consider both the advantages and risks associated with this treatment.

---

37 Brandeis, J., Lu, S. and Runels, C. (2024) '(229) a pilot study of a novel PRP protocol to increase penile length, girth, and function', The Journal of Sexual Medicine, 21(Supplement_1). doi:10.1093/jsxmed/qdae001.219.

38 https://academic.oup.com/jsm/article/21/Supplement_1/ qdae001.219/7600882

39 Penile BOTOX injections improve blood flow and other outcomes in men with moderate to severe erectile dysfunction | HTB | HIV i-Base https://i-base.info/htb/45217

Benefits of Botox Penile Injections

One of the primary benefits of Botox injections in the penile area is the improvement of blood flow. A study has indicated that Botox treatment can improve blood flow to the penis to help with ED. However, it also can lead to harder, more full erections[40]. Additionally, there is evidence suggesting that Botox injections may modestly increase stretched penile length. A man can expect to see an increase in length from a single Botox injection between 0.4-0.8 inches (about 1-2 centimeters). The shaft of the penis also expands as the body responds to the Botox to potentially increase girth.

Risks of Botox Penile Injection

Using Botox injections for growth are an off-label use as seen in other cosmetic treatments and haven't yet been approved by the FDA. However, side effects are minimal. In one study, they found that side effects for Botox Penile Injections are relatively low at a rate of 4%, which were mostly some bruising and acute pain after the injection that eventually went away. These effects are on par with using Botox injections on your face.

A study on the long-term effectiveness and safety of Botox for ED treatment by the National Institutes of Health suggests that the preliminary evidence supports its use and that more research is needed[41].

40   https://i-base.info/htb/45217
41   https://pubmed.ncbi.nlm.nih.gov/34937674/

SURGICAL PENILE ENLARGEMENT — IMPLANTS FOR LENGTH AND GIRTH

Is penile enlargement surgery right for you? Surgery is typically recommended only as a last resort. Why? After over two decades of being a urologist, my opinion is that nothing is as good as a natural erection. Even if it's induced with medications or injections, the quality of a natural erection is the best. If a patient fails to respond to all prior therapies, then we can consider placing an inflatable penile implant for a gentleman. The procedure is relatively simple. The operation takes about 1.5 to two hours to perform, and it's typically an outpatient procedure. After recuperation, the penile implant can be activated.

Benefits of Penis Enlargement Surgery:

1. Increased size: the primary benefit sought from penis enlargement surgery is an increase in the length or girth of the penis, which can be achieved with an implant or inflatable device. This physical change can lead to greater self-esteem and confidence in some men.

2. Permanent solution: unlike temporary measures such as the use of extenders or pumps, surgical enlargement offers a permanent solution to size concerns.

3. Psychological well-being: for men with severe anxiety or psychological distress due to their perception of having a small penis, surgery may provide a psychological benefit and improve their quality of life.

Risks of Penis Enlargement Surgery with an Implant

1. Infection: as with any surgical procedure, there is a risk of infection. This can be more concerning with an implant, as the introduction of a foreign body into the penis increases the risk.

2. Implant issues: there is a possibility of implant breakage or malfunction over time, which may require additional surgeries to address.

3. Scarring and disfigurement: surgery can lead to scarring, which might cause the penis to become disfigured. In some cases, this can lead to a decrease in penis size or a change in its shape.

4. Sensory changes: there is a risk of reduced sensitivity in the penis, which can affect sexual pleasure.

Risks of Penis Enlargement Surgery with an Inflatable Device

1. Mechanical failure: inflatable devices can suffer from mechanical problems, necessitating further surgery to repair or replace the device.

2. Erosion: over time, the device may erode through the skin or into the urethra, which can be painful and may require surgical correction.

HOW INFLATABLE DEVICES WORK

Each time that a patient wants to get a full erection, he presses a button that will inflate the prosthesis, thereby creating an erection. In our experience, a natural erection is typically longer and wider than the erection induced by an inflatable penile implant. However, when all else fails, the penile implant can be a great solution for a man without other good options. The implants are typically good for several years, and the duration and longevity vary from a few years up to 10 years per implant. The benefits of an implant include that the patient can achieve an erection whenever he wants and as long as he chooses, creating somewhat of a Superman phenomenon during sexual activity. We would rather support a man to develop normal erections, but if all else fails, a penile implant can be a suitable solution.

LIGAMENTOLYSIS: SURGERY TO INCREASE PENIS LENGTH

Ligamentolysis surgery, also known as penile suspensory ligament division, is a procedure aimed at treating a condition known as "buried penis," which can also have the effect of increasing perceived penis length. The suspensory ligament that connects your penis to your pubic bone is surgically cut. The flaccid penis hangs lower and seems longer. The surgery involves cutting the ligament that attaches the penis to the pubic bone, allowing more of the shaft to hang outside the body, which can give the appearance of increased length, particularly in the flaccid state. This procedure does not affect the length of the penis in the erect state.

Benefits of Ligamentolysis:

- Aesthetic improvement: for men with a buried penis, the surgery can improve the cosmetic appearance of the genitalia, making the penis more visible.
- Functional enhancement: it can potentially improve sexual function and comfort by releasing the penis from the pubic bone and allowing better access during sexual activity.
- Psychological impact: the procedure may enhance self-esteem and body image in men who are self-conscious about the size of their penis.

Risks of Ligamentolysis:

- Surgical complications: as with any surgical procedure, there is a risk of infection, bleeding, and adverse reactions to anesthesia.

- Scarring: there may be scarring at the site of the incision, which can effect the appearance or function of the penis.
- Altered sensation: some men may experience altered sensation or decreased sensitivity in the penis following the surgery.
- Instability: the penis may become less stable when erect, as the suspensory ligament provides support during an erection.
- Unsatisfactory results: not all patients will be satisfied with the results, and perceived increases in length may not meet expectations. For these gentlemen, I offer penile injections for growth options.

Men considering this surgery should have a thorough discussion with their surgeon about the potential risks and benefits, and realistic expectations should be set. It is also important to consider that non-surgical alternatives for buried penis, such as weight loss or therapy, may be recommended before considering ligamentolysis.

8.   Scrotox - Scrotum Botox Injections

A growing trend in male enhancement is Scrotox, which are Botox injections into the scrotum to smooth out wrinkles and reduce sweating. It was originally explored as an option for testicular pain relief; however, other benefits were discovered. As the scrotum reacts to the Botox injections, it expands to reduce wrinkles. It also tightens sweat pores to reduce the amount of sweat secreted.

BENEFITS OF SCROTOX:

- Reduction in sweating: hyperhidrosis, or excessive sweating, can be an uncomfortable and embarrassing condition that can affect the scrotal area. Scrotox has been reported to decrease sweating in the groin area, which can contribute to a reduction in discomfort and the prevention of associated skin irritation or infections.

- Improvement in comfort: the relaxation of the dartos muscle in the scrotum, which is responsible for the wrinkling and contraction of the scrotal skin, can lead to testicles hanging lower. This can result in decreased tightness and a potential increase in comfort, especially during physical activities or in warmer climates.

- Reduced testicular pain: the same relaxation effect in the smooth muscles in the scrotum may bring pain relief to those experiencing testicular pain. Always see a urologist first if you have this symptom to get an accurate diagnosis[42].

- Potential sexual benefits: although not as widely studied, there are anecdotal reports that Scrotox may lead to improved sexual experiences. By reducing sweating and making the scrotal skin less tight, it is thought that sensitivity may be enhanced, potentially improving sexual pleasure. More research is needed.

---

42   https://pubmed.ncbi.nlm.nih.gov/25284738/

COSMETIC CIRCUMCISION

Cosmetic circumcision for adults refers to the surgical removal of the foreskin from the penis primarily for aesthetic reasons rather than for medical or religious ones. This procedure is performed by a qualified surgeon and can be done using various techniques to achieve the desired cosmetic outcome.

The benefits of cosmetic circumcision can include:

- Aesthetic preferences: some men choose to undergo circumcision for personal aesthetic preferences, desiring a penis appearance that is consistent with circumcised norms within certain cultures or societies. A study has shown that patients and their partners may be more satisfied with the aesthetic result of circumcision (PMC).
- Hygiene: circumcision can make it easier to maintain genital hygiene as it eliminates the foreskin, which can sometimes harbor bacteria and other pathogens. While proper hygiene can be maintained without circumcision, some men may find it simpler to keep the area clean without the foreskin[43].
- Potential reduction in infection risk: some studies suggest that circumcised men may have a lower risk of certain sexually transmitted infections (STIs), including HIV. However, it's important to note that safe sex practices are crucial regardless of circumcision status.
- Reduced risk of certain medical conditions: adult circumcision may reduce the risk of developing conditions such as phimosis (tightness of the foreskin that prevents its retraction over the glans) and balanitis (inflammation of the glans). The procedure can be especially useful in patients who have phimosis[44].

---

43 https://www.mayoclinic.org/tests-procedures/circumcision/about/
    pac-20393550
44 https://www.ncbi.nlm.nih.gov/pmc/articles/PMC8072165/

While there are potential benefits, circumcision is a personal decision and the perceived benefits can vary greatly. Men considering this procedure should discuss the risks and benefits with a qualified healthcare provider to make an informed decision.

PART III

YOUR PROSTATE

The prostate is an essential gland that plays a role in ejaculation and orgasms. The prostate supplies the semen, which combines with the sperm produced by the testicles in order to deliver the sperm during ejaculation. It's connected to a network of nerves that are connected to the penis and can play a role in the orgasm process. This is why surgical removal of part or all of the prostate can impact your ability to orgasm if the nerves are severed during the surgery.

Blood flow can become problematic in the spongy tissue of the prostate, which doesn't have as much blood flow as the penis or the testicles. When blood stagnates, it slows down the immune response to infections as well as the healing process via platelets. Over time, prostates are more likely to become inflamed or enlarged, which can cause urinary incontinence and erectile dysfunction.

Your primary care physician and urologist will test for your PSA (Prostate Specific Antigen) every year after age 40. This can be an early indicator of prostate cancer, which is why screening is so important, as earlier treatment is more effective and has fewer side effects than more advanced-stage prostate cancer. Since prostate cancer is the second leading cause of cancer death among US men and one in eight men will have prostate cancer in their lifetime, we need to talk about optimizing sexual health for prostate cancer survivors[45].

---

45 https://www.cancer.org/cancer/types/prostate-cancer/about/key-statistics.
   html

9. Prostate Cancer – The Impact on Sexual Performance

Prostate cancer itself, as well as certain prostate cancer treatments, can cause ED. We see a lot of men who are concerned about having cancer, developing cancer, and if they have cancer, what's the best way for them to be treated? Many of my patients have confessed that they are more afraid of the side effects of treatment, such as ED or urinary incontinence, than they are of the prostate cancer itself. This fear of losing the normal functions of their penis deters many male patients from getting their PSA checked, especially after 40.

However, patients that are afraid of the side effects will find relief in knowing that we've made major advancements in the selective treatment of prostate cancer. The advanced technologies used at Comprehensive Urology, are able to correctly diagnose and more precisely identify the locations of the cancers. We can also target the prostate cancer cells while preserving as many healthy cells as possible so that the prostate continues to function even after treatment. In the past, the man could only have removal of the prostate or radiation in the prostate. We're able to now identify where the cancer is located, take care of it as an outpatient treatment, and thereby preserve and maximize preservation of the normal sexual and urinary function. Thanks to the advanced technologies and expertise that we have at Comprehensive Urology, we can provide a completely new way of looking at urological conditions and diagnosing and treating them.

There are two things to remember for prostate cancer patients who either have ED or want to prevent it:

1. There are minimally invasive therapies to treat prostate cancer in a targeted way with less side effects than prostatectomy (surgically removing part or all of the prostate).
2. Prehabilitation works! Prehabilitation is prophylactic treatment before a prostate cancer procedure, such as robotic surgery or focal therapy (HIFU, TULSA).

10. Minimally Invasive Prostate Cancer Treatments to Preserve Erectile Function

Since prostate cancer treatment can increase the chances of having ED, the choice of which treatment to undergo should be carefully considered. The gold standard for advanced prostate cancer is to surgically remove the prostate (prostatectomy) in combination with other cancer treatments like radiation, hormone blockade therapy, and chemotherapy. Removing the entire prostate raises the risk of having ED substantially, which is why I save that option as a last resort. There are many other, newer prostate cancer treatments that are less invasive, and preliminary evidence indicates there may be fewer side effects.

Let's take a look at the latest options that may help you preserve your sexual performance for years to come.

WHAT'S FOCAL THERAPY FOR PROSTATE CANCER?

I was an early adopter of Focal Therapy for prostate cancer, which covers a series of techniques that use energy, heat, and freezing to target prostate cancer cells in a more focused way. Hence, the name Focal Therapy.

In the state of California, I've performed more Focal Therapy procedures (HIFU and TULSA-Pro combined) than any other surgeon as of 2023. I'm also involved in cutting-edge research for this next generation of prostate cancer treatments. So the information I share with you comes both from new research as well as my own experience as a pioneering surgeon.

With Focal Therapies, we're now able to identify where prostate cancer is located using live MRI's and use high-intensity ultrasound to target cancer cells. If you're a candidate for Focal Therapy, you can avoid surgery, avoid radiation, all while maintaining a higher level of normal sexual function and bladder integrity. It's been a game changer for many men with prostate cancer.

In the past, surgery was the main tool for removing tumors from the prostate, or for removing the entire prostate completely. However, the incidence of ED is at a rate of after the standard of care, a radical prostatectomy (removal of the entire prostate) is 85%.[46] For patients with stage 2 or 3 prostate cancer, we now have two focal therapies to choose from: HIFU and TULSA. HIFU's ED rates are at 37%.[47] Tulsa has been found to have even fewer side effects than prostatectomy with an ED rate of only 23%.[48]

So, the first step to preserving erectile function in prostate cancer patients is to choose the most minimally invasive therapy that is the appropriate choice for their individual case. I try to preserve as much of the healthy prostate as possible, and focal therapies allow me two choices on how to treat the prostate cancer cells in a more targeted way. Prostate surgery is always an option down the road if the cancer shows up again. Long story short, I save the most radical options for

---

46   https://www.ncbi.nlm.nih.gov/pmc/articles/PMC5005072/
47   https://www.ncbi.nlm.nih.gov/pmc/articles/PMC5005072/
48   https://pubmed.ncbi.nlm.nih.gov/33021440/

last whenever possible. Sometimes, surgery is the best option, but if there's a chance of treatment without surgery, I recommend that my patients consider focal therapy.

WHAT IS HIFU FOR PROSTATE CANCER?

High-Intensity Focused Ultrasound (HIFU) is a minimally invasive treatment option for prostate cancer that uses focused ultrasound waves to heat and destroy cancerous tissue in the prostate. This technology targets only the affected areas, aiming to minimize damage to surrounding healthy tissue.

Benefits of HIFU

- Minimally invasive: HIFU is less invasive than traditional surgical options, which can lead to quicker recovery times.
- Preservation of quality of life: studies have shown that HIFU has lower risks of urinary incontinence and erectile dysfunction compared to more invasive treatments like surgery or radiation.
- Outpatient procedure: HIFU is often performed on an outpatient basis, allowing patients to go home the same day[49].

Risks of HIFU

- Incomplete treatment: there is a risk that HIFU may not treat all the cancerous cells, potentially requiring additional treatment.
- Urinary side effects: some men may experience urinary symptoms post-treatment, such as frequency, urgency, or retention.

---

49   https://www.ncbi.nlm.nih.gov/pmc/articles/PMC7327297/

- Erectile dysfunction: while the rates are generally lower than with radical prostatectomy, erectile dysfunction is still a potential risk following HIFU treatment. Studies suggest that erectile function outcomes are better with HIFU than with more invasive treatments, but this can vary based on individual cases[50].

ERECTILE DYSFUNCTION RATES

The rates of erectile dysfunction after HIFU vary between studies, but they are generally considered to be lower than those associated with radical prostatectomy. The exact rate of ED can depend on several factors, including the patient's age, baseline erectile function, and the extent of the area treated. Prehabilitation with Shockwave Therapy may be an option to preserve ED if done before the procedure and potentially afterward.

WHAT IS THE TULSA PROCEDURE
FOR PROSTATE CANCER?

The TULSA procedure, which stands for Transurethral Ultrasound Ablation, is a minimally invasive treatment for prostate cancer that uses directional ultrasound to deliver precise doses of heat that ablate (destroy) prostate cancer cells. I perform this outpatient procedure with real-time MRI guidance to target cancerous tissue while sparing as much of the surrounding healthy tissues as possible. TULSA allows me to minimize side effects by preserving as much of the healthy parts of the prostate as possible.

---

50   https://www.mayoclinic.org/medical-professionals/urology/news/high-intensity-focused-ultrasound-for-the-treatment-of-prostate-cancer/mqc-20519431

TULSA is an outpatient procedure that is done at a radiology center as you will be inside an MRI machine, so I can view the cancer in your prostate live. A small device is inserted into the urethra like a catheter. Once we map out the cancer in your prostate, we begin the heating phase of the treatment, which typically takes under an hour. You leave the same day.

It's important to note that I am an investigator on the Captain Study, a phase 3 clinical trial that is studying to see how effective the TULSA Procedure is compared to standard treatment. Since this is an active study, we can't report the results yet until it's finished. Results will be available here when the study is published: https://comprehensive-urology.com/clinical-trials/

What I can share is that the Captain study will also help us determine the prevalence of side effects after the procedure, including TULSA's impact on erectile function and bladder continence. It will also be used to further validate the safety of the procedure when compared to the previously completed study. A full summary of the ongoing study can be found here:

https://www.urologytimes.com/view/tulsa-compared-with-radical-prostatectomy-in-phase-3-trial

However, I can share the results of a previous TULSA-Pro study called the TACT study, which led to the FDA approving the TULSA procedure for use in prostate cancer. It found that TULSA-Pro reduced the PSA of 95% of study participants, 65% didn't have any evidence of cancer 12 months later, and 75% either maintained their current erectile function or regained function after the procedure. This study prompted researchers to further compare TULSA to both the more established HIFU Focal Therapy, and the standard of care, surgery.

Reasons why TULSA-Pro has gained so much attention:

- Targeted treatment: MRI guidance allows for precise targeting of the prostate tissue, reducing the likelihood of damaging nearby tissues and organs.
- High preservation of sexual function: there is a high rate of preserving erectile function post-procedure.
- Minimally invasive: the procedure is done transurethrally, which means a device is inserted like a catheter to heat targeted areas of the prostate, so it's less invasive than traditional surgery.
- Outpatient procedure: you leave the same day. TULSA-pro typically has a quicker recovery time compared to surgery.

Risks for TULSA-Pro:

- Urinary symptoms: some patients may experience urinary symptoms post-treatment, including urgency, frequency, or retention. 2.6% had urinary incontinence, and 2.6% had urethral stricture.
- Erectile dysfunction: while the rates of erectile dysfunction are reportedly low, it remains a potential risk. The data collected at 2 years post-treatment indicates that TULSA-PRO has a low rate of erectile dysfunction, with 23% moderate ED (Grade 2, medication indicated)[51] This incidence of ED is significantly less than the gold standard treatment of removing part or all of the prostate gland.

---

51   https://pubmed.ncbi.nlm.nih.gov/33021440/

WHAT IS PREHABILITATION BEFORE
PROSTATE CANCER TREATMENT?

Since many prostate cancer treatments come with the risk of erectile dysfunction, I've had many of my patients prehabilitate their penis before they go into a procedure or surgery. By using Shockwave Therapy in the months before the procedure, we're able to build up the blood vessels that can preserve the circulatory health of your penis. We supercharge it so that you go into the procedure or surgery with a higher baseline erectile function.

My patients who take this extra step before the surgery are more likely to preserve their erectile function after the procedure/surgery. Post-op rehabilitation is also much easier when you prehabilitate because your body has already been conditioned to a higher level of blood circulation. Better flowing blood means less inflammation after a procedure as well as better erections.

HORMONE BLOCKADE THERAPY
FOR PROSTATE CANCER

One of the treatments employed for prostate cancer is hormone blockade therapy, also known as androgen deprivation therapy (ADT). Since prostate cancer can grow more quickly from testosterone and related androgens, the idea behind blockade therapy is to deprive prostate cancer of these hormones in the hopes of reducing the prostate cancer's ability to grow. Hormone blockade therapy is a treatment designed to reduce levels of male hormones, or androgens, in the body, with the primary androgen being testosterone. Prostate cancer cells usually require testosterone to grow and proliferate. By lowering testosterone levels or blocking its effects, hormone blockade therapy can slow down or even shrink the growth of prostate cancer.

METHODS OF HORMONE BLOCKADE THERAPY

- Luteinizing Hormone-Releasing Hormone (LHRH) Agonists: these drugs reduce the amount of testosterone produced by the testicles.
- LHRH antagonists: similar to LHRH agonists, these prevent the testicles from receiving messages to make testosterone.
- Anti-androgens: these medications block testosterone from binding to prostate cancer cells.
- Orchiectomy: a surgical procedure that involves the removal of the testicles to drastically reduce the production of testosterone.

Benefits of Blockage Therapy

- Delay the progression of prostate cancer: especially beneficial in advanced stages of the disease.
- Reduce symptoms: in cases where cancer has spread, hormone therapy can help relieve symptoms, such as bone pain.
- Shrink the tumor: this can be particularly useful before radiation therapy or surgery.
- Increase survival rates: When used in conjunction with other treatments, hormone therapy can improve overall survival for some men with prostate cancer.

Risks of Blockade Therapy

- Hot flashes: a common side effect similar to those experienced by women during menopause.
- Reduced sexual function and desire: due to the lowered testosterone levels.
- Loss of bone density (osteoporosis): this can increase the risk of fractures.
- Weight gain and muscle loss: changes in body composition can occur that feminizes the masculine physique.

11. BPH – Benign Prostatic Hyperplasia

Reducing the size of the prostate for people with benign prostate hyperplasia (a.k.a. enlarged prostate) can reduce symptoms such as interruptions in urinary stream, incontinence, and ED. The question becomes, what is the best way to reduce the size of your prostate for you?

MEDICATION FOR BPH TREATMENT

Finasteride is a medication that is usually used in a 1 mg dose to stop male pattern baldness and regrow hair. It works by blocking the conversion of testosterone to dihydrotestosterone (DHT), which is the hormone that triggers hair loss.

At a dosage of 5 mg, finasteride has been clinically proven to be an effective treatment for reducing the symptoms of BPH. In clinical trials, finasteride has been shown to improve urinary symptom scores more significantly than placebo, especially in trials lasting more than one year. It works by inhibiting the enzyme 5-alpha-reductase, which is responsible for converting testosterone to DHT, a hormone that contributes to prostate growth.

CLINICAL TRIAL FINDINGS:

- Symptom improvement: finasteride has consistently improved urinary symptom scores, indicating a reduction in the severity of BPH symptoms

- Reduced risk of BPH progression: the treatment has been found to significantly lower the risk of BPH progression, meaning that it can help prevent the worsening of the condition over time[52]
- Decreased prostate volume: finasteride has been effective in decreasing the overall size of the prostate, which is directly correlated with the severity of BPH symptoms[53]

The use of finasteride 5 mg is well-established and has a strong safety profile for the treatment of men with BPH. It is an important option for men seeking a non-surgical approach to managing their BPH symptoms. However, patients should be aware that finasteride may take several months to show maximal effects, and continued use is typically necessary to maintain symptom relief. It's also important to note that while finasteride can reduce the overall risk of urinary retention and the need for BPH-related surgery, it does come with potential side effects, such as sexual dysfunction, which should be discussed with a healthcare provider.

There are other medications that can help with BPH symptoms, but don't actually treat the condition itself. Medications used to manage the symptoms of Benign Prostatic Hyperplasia (BPH) typically fall into the following categories:

1. Alpha Blockers: these medications relax the muscles of the bladder neck and prostate, making it easier to urinate. Commonly prescribed alpha blockers include:
   - Alfuzosin (Uroxatral)
   - Doxazosin (Cardura)
   - Prazosin (Minipress)
   - Silodosin (Rapaflo)
   - Tamsulosin (Flomax)
   - Terazosin (Hytrin)

---

52 https://www.ncbi.nlm.nih.gov/pmc/articles/PMC8908761/
53 https://www.nejm.org/doi/full/10.1056/NEJM199210223271701

2. 5-alpha Reductase Inhibitors: these drugs shrink the prostate by preventing hormonal changes that cause prostate growth. Examples include:
    - Finasteride (Proscar)
    - Dutasteride (Avodart)

3. Phosphodiesterase-5 Inhibitors: this class of drugs, represented by tadalafil (Cialis), is traditionally used to treat erectile dysfunction but can also help BPH symptoms by relaxing muscles in the bladder and prostate.

4. Combination therapy: for some men, a combination of an alpha-blocker and a 5-alpha reductase inhibitor is more effective than either drug alone.

BUTTERFLY CLINICAL TRIAL FOR THOSE WHO FAILED HORMONE BLOCKADE THERAPY

There's a small device that can be placed through the urethra that can help with symptoms of BPH. Primarily, this device can help with maintaining a healthy urinary stream with less incidence of urinary incontinence. It has also been shown to help maintain erectile function as well as improve it in men who were previously not sexually active[54].

I'm currently part of a new study to further explore how this device can help men who failed Hormone Blockade Therapy. If you'd like to learn more about the Butterfly Device Clinical study, please visit: https://comprehensive-urology.com/clinical-trials/

---

54 https://www.ncbi.nlm.nih.gov/pmc/articles/PMC10129019/

REZŪM WATER THERAPY

Rezūm water vapor therapy is a minimally invasive treatment for Benign Prostatic Hyperplasia (BPH), which is an enlargement of the prostate gland that can cause urinary difficulties. This therapy uses water vapor (steam) to deliver targeted, controlled doses of thermal energy directly to the prostate tissue, causing cell death and reducing the size of the gland.

Benefits of Rezūm:

- Minimally invasive: Rezūm is less invasive compared to traditional surgical options like transurethral resection of the prostate (TURP), leading to a quicker recovery (NCBI).
- Preservation of sexual function: the treatment has a lower risk of sexual dysfunction compared to some other BPH treatments (NCBI).
- Short procedure time: the procedure can be performed in a short time, often under 30 minutes, and usually under sedation or local anesthesia.
- Outpatient procedure: typically done as an outpatient procedure, allowing patients to return home the same day.

Risks of Rezūm:

- Urinary symptoms: some men may experience temporary urinary side effects such as urgency, discomfort, or the need for catheterization shortly after the procedure.
- Infection: as with any procedure, there is a risk of urinary tract infection or prostatitis.
- Need for retreatment: while many men experience long-term relief, some may

require additional treat-
ment if symptoms return[55].

UROLIFT

The UroLift® system is a minimally invasive treatment for Benign
Prostatic Hyperplasia (BPH), which is an enlargement of the prostate
gland causing urinary symptoms. This procedure involves the placement
of small implants to lift and hold the enlarged prostate tissue out of
the way, thereby relieving obstruction of the urethra without cutting,
heating, or removing prostate tissue.

Benefits of UroLift

- Rapid symptom relief:
  patients often experience
  improvement in BPH
  symptoms quickly after the
  procedure (NCBI).
- Preservation of sexual
  function: UroLift® is
  designed to preserve
  sexual function, a significant advantage over some
  other BPH treatments that
  can lead to sexual dysfunction (NCBI).
- Minimally invasive: the
  procedure is less invasive
  than traditional surgical
  options, typically resulting
  in a shorter recovery time.
- Outpatient procedure: it
  is usually performed on
  an outpatient basis, which
  means patients can go
  home the same day.

Risks of UroLift

- Temporary urinary
  symptoms: some men
  may experience tempo-
  rary urinary discomfort,
  urgency, or blood in
  the urine following the
  procedure.

---

55   https://www.ncbi.nlm.nih.gov/pmc/articles/PMC6180381/

- Need for retreatment:
  although many men have
  long-lasting relief, some
  may eventually require
  additional treatment for
  BPH symptoms.

- Rare complications: as with
  any medical procedure,
  there are risks of rare but
  serious complications
  such as infection or device
  malfunction.

AQUABLATION

Aquablation therapy is a novel treatment for Benign Prostatic Hyperplasia (BPH), which utilizes a high-velocity waterjet to remove prostate tissue. This procedure is robotically executed and guided by real-time ultrasound imaging, allowing for precise removal of the enlarged prostate tissue that causes urinary symptoms.

Benefits of Aquablation

- Precision: the combination
  of real-time imaging and
  robotic execution allows
  for precise targeting of
  prostate tissue, which can
  improve outcomes (NCBI).
- Suitable for various
  prostate sizes: Aquablation
  has been shown to be
  effective for a wide range
  of prostate sizes, including
  very large prostates (NCBI).
- Preservation of sexual
  function: the procedure
  aims to preserve sexual
  function, which is a significant concern for many
  patients undergoing BPH
  treatment.
- Consistent outcomes:
  because the procedure
  is robotically executed, it
  may offer more consistent
  outcomes than those
  dependent on manual
  surgical techniques.

Risks of Aquablation

- Bleeding: one of the most
  significant risks associated with Aquablation

- is bleeding, which may require further intervention or blood transfusion.
- Urinary symptoms: post-operative irritation can cause urinary symptoms such as urgency, frequency, or the need for temporary catheterization.
- Need for additional treatment: as with other BPH treatments, there is a possibility that not all symptomatic tissue will be removed, or that symptoms will recur, necessitating additional treatment[56].

12. Shockwave Therapy for your Prostate

The prostate gland is about the size of a walnut and is located behind the penis, sitting just above the space between your legs. That space between the scrotum and the anus is called the perineum, which encompasses the skin and membranes just below your prostate. These membranes are thin enough that we can send low-intensity sound waves, using Shockwave Therapy, into the prostate from outside the body by putting the nozzle of the device on the perineum. Since the sound waves increase blood flow to the area, it's useful for symptoms that result from inflammation of the prostate.

Inflammatory conditions of the prostate include:

- Chronic prostatitis (prostatitis without a bacterial infection)
- BPH (Benign Prostatic Hyperplasia)
- Pelvic pain related to an enlarged prostate
- Decreased urinary flow due to enlarged prostate

---

56   https://www.ncbi.nlm.nih.gov/pmc/articles/PMC6373984/

When we started to notice the benefits of low-intensity Shockwave Therapy when used in the perineum area in addition to the penis itself, we began collective case studies to see if this could be an effective noninvasive approach to symptoms associated with inflamed or enlarged prostates. Using sound waves the same way we are able to use that modality to get rid of inflammatory conditions and other body parts, we can do the same thing for the prostate. So, men who have chronic prostatitis not due to bacteria can get significant relief with the use of low-intensity Shockwave Therapy in the perineum.

Please visit https://comprehensive-urology.com/clinical-trials/ to find out more about our active observational studies using Shockwave Therapy.

PART IV

YOUR TESTOSTERONE

13. Understanding Testosterone

Testosterone is a key hormone that helps develop male characteristics and sexual organs. Embryos by default will have female genitalia: clitoris and labia (as well as a vagina, and fallopian tubes). Embryos that experience higher testosterone levels will transform their genitalia to a male form: the clitoris and corporal bodies elongate to become a penis and the labia fuse

to create a scrotum. In adults, testosterone is the hormone that at higher levels creates male characteristics such as facial and body hair, deeper voice, and larger muscle and bone mass and is integral to the development of normal sexual characteristics. Testosterone is, however, much more than just a sex hormone. It is integral to a normal, healthy body and brain.

Testosterone Replacement Therapy (TRT) is often prescribed to men who have been diagnosed with hypogonadism, a condition where the body does not produce enough testosterone. Clinical results of TRT have shown several potential benefits, particularly in sexual function, among other aspects of health and quality of life.

SEXUAL FUNCTION IMPROVEMENTS WITH TRT:

- Libido: TRT has been consistently shown to improve libido or sexual desire in men with low testosterone levels.
- Erectile function: many studies have reported improvements in erectile function with TRT, although results can vary based on the individual and the severity of erectile dysfunction before treatment.
- Overall sexual satisfaction: an increase in overall sexual satisfaction has been observed in some men undergoing TRT.

- Other clinical results:
- Mood and quality of life: some men report improvement in mood and a sense of well-being after starting TRT.
- Body composition: TRT may help increase lean body mass and decrease fat mass in men with low testosterone.
- Bone density: there is evidence that TRT can increase bone density, which is beneficial in preventing osteoporosis.

However, TRT is not without risks and is a subject of ongoing research and debate. Potential risks include an increased likelihood of developing cardiovascular issues, sleep apnea, and prostate abnormalities. The therapy should only be initiated after a thorough evaluation by a healthcare provider, and men on TRT require regular monitoring to manage any potential side effects and to adjust treatment as necessary.

Increasing testosterone, both naturally, and through replacement therapy can revive your energy, mood, and mental clarity. Here are some of the benefits I've noticed firsthand in patients who had low T and increased testosterone:

- Sharper thinking: many men with low T feel that they have mental fog, can't recall names or information as readily, or they feel like their mind is working slower than what they are used to.
- Balanced mood: many men with low T feel depressed, have increased anxiety, or both. We have treated many men with low T that after their testosterone was normalized they came off of their antidepressants completely and their low T had been initially misdiagnosed as depression.
- Improved libido: many men with low T present with a lowered sex drive (libido)—oftentimes this can be reversed with testosterone optimization.
- Stronger erections: many men with low T notice that their erections get stronger after their testosterone levels are optimized.

- Improved energy: many men with low T feel that they get tired sooner, need to take naps, can't recover as quickly after workouts or don't have the drive to be as active in general. Once optimized, many men can regain these normal functions and increased states of energy. Increased overall physical activity can improve overall cardiovascular health, including blood flow to the penis.
- Improved muscle mass: normal testosterone levels are key for maintaining normal muscle mass and skin appearance. With an active lifestyle, most men are able to regain muscle mass with testosterone optimization.
- Improved bone health: low T can accelerate bone loss in men and can be a risk factor for bone fractures due to osteoporosis.
- Improved metabolism: when T levels are normalized, many men notice that their blood sugar levels and their lipid profiles (cholesterol and triglyceride levels) improve! Improved metabolism can improve overall cardiovascular health, including blood flow to the penis.

HOW IS TESTOSTERONE CREATED?

The brain (in the pituitary gland) releases a compound called LH (Luteinizing hormone). When released, LH stimulates the testicles to make testosterone. Testosterone is then created but most of it is bound to large proteins in the bloodstream. This "bound" testosterone is too large to enter cells and is therefore "not active." The testosterone that is not bound to proteins (free testosterone) can enter cells and is active, as are testosterone molecules bound to small proteins. Hence, the bioactive levels of T (free T and T bound to small proteins) are the key levels to check and monitor when evaluating a man for low T or T optimization.

WHAT ARE NORMAL T LEVELS?

The key levels are the bioavailable levels of T. The range for normal is quite broad. Therefore, if a man is in the normal or low normal range of bioavailable T, he may still benefit from T optimization.

The highest T levels occur in the morning hours (a key reason why healthy men get morning erections), so it is best to check T levels in the morning (preferably between 8-10 AM).

HOW CAN I NATURALLY IMPROVE MY T LEVELS?

1. Get adequate, good-quality sleep.
2. Stress management; do things that make you happy.
3. Weight training (in particular the larger muscle groups in the body, such as thighs and buttock muscles).
4. Avoid excessive alcohol.
5. Losing excessive fat (try to get down to your ideal body mass).

TRT DELIVERY METHODS

There are multiple ways to replace T in your body: pills, gels, nasal sprays, injections, and pellets. But which method is best for you and is T replacement therapy right for you?

For you to determine if testosterone replacement therapy is right for you, you need to make sure that with every method you choose, you are able to get adequate levels consistently.

In our experience, we find that T injections are the most effective way to determine if T therapy is of clinical benefit to our patients. A simple way to start is to get a T injection once a week for 8 weeks and monitor your clinical symptoms.

Here are the questions to track your response:

1. How is my brain working? Do I feel sharper? Am I able to process information better, and faster? Is my memory improving?
2. How is my mood? Do I feel happier, do I feel more positive, do I have less anxiety? Am I sleeping better?
3. How is my energy level: do I feel more energy? Do I fatigue less? Do I recover from workouts better or faster?
4. How has my sex drive improved?
5. Are my erections stronger? Am I getting morning erections now? Do I sustain my erection for a longer time?
6. Has my ejaculatory volume increased?
7. Is it easier to build muscle mass? Do I feel stronger?

If you find that any of these parameters improve for you significantly, then T therapy can be right for you.

TRT SIDE EFFECTS

The side effects of T replacement appear to be limited. The main ones include:

1. For about 5% of men, red blood cell size can increase. In these situations, we look to change the formulation or route of delivery, and sometimes, men will have to donate blood to lower their blood count back to normal.
2. In some men, their estrogen levels also increase with their T levels—for these men, we either lower their T dose or give them

supplements (like zinc or DIM) or medications to keep their estrogen levels in a normal range.

3.   Rarely, some men mention that they get:

- Acne: can be treated with topical medicine
- Hair loss: can be prevented in some men with medications
- Shorter-fused: we look to change the dose, route, or frequency of the T therapy

WHAT ABOUT THE RISK OF PROSTATE CANCER ON TESTOSTERONE?

In the past, this was a concern, however, more recent scientific evidence does not show a correlation between T therapy and developing prostate cancer. So prostate cancer survivors and patients in treatment can receive Testosterone Replacement Therapy TRT.[57] Some men who have undergone treatment for prostate cancer are actually placed on TRT as part of their recovery.

WHAT ABOUT FERTILITY AND TESTOSTERONE?

Suppose a man wants to increase his testosterone but wants to preserve his fertility. In that case, we strongly encourage that person to bank some sperm at a baseline, then use medications to stimulate his own production of T, such as by using clomiphene citrate, or HCG and avoiding taking T injections, or T replacement meds.

If these oral pills work so well, why not use them as the first line in treating all men with low T? After the initial eight weeks, if we see that

---

57   https://www.ncbi.nlm.nih.gov/pmc/articles/PMC6392157/

a man responds favorably to T therapy, then we discuss the different modes of therapy. For younger men or men who want to preserve their fertility, we recommend these medications (clomiphene or HCG). In older men, these medications often do not provide the same clinical benefits as T replacement therapy, so we use a combination of T replacement therapies in conjunction with either clomiphene citrate or HCG.

WILL I BECOME DEPENDENT ON T THERAPY?

Men who are lacking T get on T therapy. Therefore, it is highly likely (but not always the case) that most men will need to stay on T therapy. A key consideration that many health care providers forget is that if a patient is placed on T replacement therapy, the body gets fooled into believing it has ample T levels. The testicles start to produce less on their own and, over time, can shrink in size. For this reason, we strongly recommend that men be placed on either clomiphene citrate or HCG when being placed on long-term T replacement therapy. With this approach, we can better preserve a man's own natural T production capacity and testicular volume.

A LOW TESTOSTERONE TREATMENT SUCCESS STORY

One of the most memorable stories about TRT that I have is of a gentleman who came in to see us in a wheelchair. He was a young man in his early 30s diagnosed with multiple sclerosis. He came to us for a urological need because he felt that he may have low testosterone. He had been to many different practitioners who have told them that his testosterone levels are within a normal range. The problem is that the range for testosterone is so wide, typically between 300 to about a thousand. And in that realm, there's so much possibility for improvement. So they told him, "No, you're not a candidate." We took a look and said, "You know what? We feel that based on our experience that we've had with patients, you definitely have room for improvement."

We started a mono testing replacement protocol. After about two months of him being monitored by us, he said, "I'm beginning to move the little toe on my foot." We continued his therapy because he was feeling better overall. And then a few months later, he came in on crutches. I asked, "What happened to your wheelchair?" He was regaining the ability to move his legs. We saw him a few months later, and he was walking on two feet with no assistance. Then we started to get pictures of him skydiving, doing as many adventures as he possibly could. He was now living an incredibly full life.

This was about 15 years ago. He is still fully functional, active, vibrant, and appreciative of his life. Every time we see him, the hugs that are exchanged and the "thank yous" that are exchanged are incredible. There's nothing more rewarding than that.

It's interesting how many patients have been diagnosed with depression. They're not all depressed. They have low T. We've had several patients come to us who've been on SSRIs for a long period of time. They come to see us and as part of our workup, we take a look at a full panel of their hormones. I can't tell you how many patients we've seen that have low T.

Based on our experience, it's worthwhile for you to try to optimize your hormones. Usually, we give an eight-week trial of T and see how you feel. I can't tell you how many people whose depression we've treated once we've optimized their testosterone.

So many of those guys get off of their antidepressant medications and live incredibly vibrant lives: energetic, happy, fulfilled, sexually active, just full of life because the right diagnosis was made for them.

Before going to a full testosterone replacement therapy, there are a few medications that could help middle-aged and older men boost their internal testosterone levels:

CLOMID

Clomiphene citrate, commonly known by its brand name Clomid, is a medication traditionally used to treat infertility in women. However, it has found off-label use in men to address issues related to low testosterone levels. Clomid works by stimulating the pituitary gland to produce more luteinizing hormone (LH) and follicle-stimulating hormone (FSH), which can increase testosterone production in the testes.

Benefits of Using Clomid to Raise Testosterone Levels

- Non-steroidal: Clomid is a non-steroidal medication, which means it does not introduce external testosterone into the body but stimulates the body's natural production.
- Improvement in hormonal balance: Clomid has been shown to effectively elevate serum testosterone levels and improve the testosterone/estrogen ratio in men with hypogonadism, which can lead to improved libido, energy levels, and mood.
- Potential fertility preservation: unlike testosterone replacement therapy, which can suppress sperm production, Clomid can preserve or even enhance fertility by increasing sperm count and quality.

- Oral administration: Clomid is convenient to take compared to testosterone injections or gels.

Risks of Using Clomid

- Side effects: potential side effects include mood swings, vision changes, and gynecomastia

- (development of breast tissue in men).
- Long-term safety uncertain: as Clomid is not FDA-approved for use in men, long-term safety data is limited.
- Varied efficacy: Clomid may not be effective for all men, and some may not respond to the treatment.

In addition to Clomid, estrogen blockers are another class of medications that can help men, particularly in the context of managing estrogen levels.

ESTROGEN BLOCKERS

Estrogen blockers, also known as aromatase inhibitors, prevent the conversion of testosterone into estrogen. Elevated estrogen levels in men can lead to various symptoms, including increased body fat, loss of muscle mass, and emotional disturbances.

Benefits of Estrogen Blockers

- Improved testosterone levels: by blocking estrogen, these medications can help maintain higher levels of testosterone.

- Reduction in estrogen-related side effects: they can mitigate issues like gynecomastia and excess fat accumulation.

Risks of Estrogen Blockers

- Bone health risks:
  long-term suppression
  of estrogen can lead to
  decreased bone density, as

While these are an option, we prefer to first try to increase the patient's natural testosterone production through lifestyle changes like improving your diet and exercise.

PART V

YOUR LIFESTYLE

14. Tony's Lifestyle Checklist for Optimal Sexual Performance

LIFESTYLE CHANGES: HEALTHY BODY, HEALTHY SEXUAL PERFORMANCE

I recommend really finding out the source of the erectile dysfunction. Are you overweight? Are you not active enough? Are you eating processed fatty foods? Are you looking at too much pornography? Are you not connected with your partner in an open relationship? Is it a vascular issue? We have things that we can test for to treat our patients better. We have vascular studies, we have blood tests, and we have the treatments all within our office to make it easier for our patients.

What are some behavioral lifestyle changes you can start to help optimize your erections?

One, if you're overweight, losing body fat makes a big difference because a lot of testosterone gets converted to estrogen by your fat cells. Having excess weight puts an encumbrance on your circulatory system. Minimize the excess weight as much as you can.

Two, take a look at your lifestyle. If it's sedentary, be much more active. The more cardiovascular health you have, the better your overall blood flow, including blood flow to your penis.

Three, how are you sleeping? If you're not getting a good night's rest, it can affect your testosterone level and indirectly your sexual function. Try to have good quality uninterrupted sleep, including having no caffeinated beverages at nighttime, minimizing alcohol in the evening hours, and minimizing drinking too much liquid. Otherwise, you may get up in the middle of the night to use the restroom and have interrupted sleep. Take a look at your stress levels.

All these things that seem cliché make a huge impact in terms of your overall health, including your sexual health.

TOP 5 STEPS FOR AN OPTIMIZED ERECTION

Some key things you can do to optimize your erection:

1. Lifestyle changes: do you have any excess body weight? Are you working out regularly? Are you getting good sleep? Are you minimizing toxins in your body, including excessive alcohol?
2. Check your testosterone level: is your testosterone level normal? Is your thyroid level normal? Is your prolactin level normal? Is your testosterone level normal?
3. Low-intensity shockwave therapies.
4. Low-dose PDE5 inhibitors can be highly effective for patients.
5. Try supplements:
   - Maca Root
   - L-Arginine
   - L-Citrulline
   - Zinc
   - Vitamin D

You can take a look at maca root, L-arginine, and L-citrulline. These are factors that can help promote nitric oxide production in your body. Zinc is a naturally occurring estrogen blocker. When we're dealing with male hormones, too much estrogen can cause excess fat, and it can decrease a man's libido and erections. Zinc is something that we use naturally in our office to help control our patient's estrogen.

Too much estrogen in the body for a male can cause fat to be placed in different areas, whether it's gynecomastia or around the belly. It's something that we check our men regularly for. Elevated estrogen levels in men can result in erectile dysfunction as well as mood disorders.

TOP 3 THINGS YOU CAN DO TO NATURALLY STIMULATE TESTOSTERONE

1. Better sleep: better sleep hygiene, no screens before bedtime, going to bed at the same time each night, waking up at the same time in the morning.
2. Physical exercise with resistance and weights: you need resistance and weights for your muscles and bones to increase your testosterone naturally.
3. Healthy diet: food is the fuel for your body, so quality fuel leads to high performance. Find out your ideal body weight. Having an excessive BMI can force your testosterone to convert into estrogen, leading to even more gains in body fat. The good news is that cutting weight stimulates testosterone levels by reducing how much is converted to estrogen.

Sleeping through the night, getting some exercise, and eating a healthier diet all lead to higher testosterone and better well-being in general.

TONY'S DIET PLAN FOR OPTIMAL SEXUAL PERFORMANCE

Diet has a considerable impact on our libido, especially when it comes to raising your testosterone naturally. To improve your testosterone at home, start by decreasing your alcohol intake. Even reducing your intake by one to two drinks a week can make a difference. Also decrease sugar intake, substituting table sugar with lower glycemic options like coconut sugar and stevia.

To obtain a better erection, we want better blood flow, and certain foods can help. The categories of foods to look for will contain:

- Nitric oxide enhancers
- Bioflavonoids
- Antioxidants

Dietary nitric oxide enhancers that will help move the blood like a rocket engine are easy to find:

- Beets
- Spinach
- Carrots
- Celery
- Lean meat
- Watermelon

Try to have one from the above list per day.

Bioflavonoids relax the blood vessels. So you can increase your intake of flavonoids by looking for dark-colored berries (blackberries and blueberries are excellent), nuts, and legumes (beans).

Let's bring it all together in a sample diet plan for a day:

Breakfast:

- Blackberry, blueberry, beet, spinach, and grass-fed whey protein smoothie
- Option for whole oats, whole grain bran, or sourdough bread

Lunch:

- Grilled salmon (high omegas can act as antioxidants and protect blood vessels)
- Spinach and green medley salad with olive oil vinaigrette
- Side of quinoa

Dinner:

- Lean poultry, baked or grilled
- Side of celery, carrots, and hummus
- Dark green vegetable of choice

Snack:

- Greek yogurt mixed with unsalted almonds or walnuts
- Side of watermelon

TONY'S LIFESTYLE CHECKLIST FOR OPTIMAL SEXUAL PERFORMANCE

1. Zinc supplements or high-zinc foods
2. Vitamin D supplements or vitamin D-rich foods
3. Cut down on fatty meals and processed foods consumption

4. Consume foods rich in omega-3 fatty acids (fish oil supplements or the Mediterranean diet)
5. Regulate your pornography consumption
6. Cardiovascular exercise
7. Weight training or resistance training
8. Get enough sleep
9. Supplements: L-arginine, L-citrulline, and Maca Root

ZINC IS AN ESTROGEN BLOCKER

Many ancient aphrodisiacs contain zinc which is one of the active ingredients in libido-boosting foods like oysters and fenugreek.

Zinc is a naturally occurring supplement that can be used to help men manage and maintain their hormones. If a male has elevated estrogen, it can cause low libido, depressive moods, and poor erections. And one thing that can be used is zinc to help block the conversion of testosterone into estrogen.

Men actually have estrogen as well as testosterone. Zinc is important to manage and balance the testosterone and estrogen ratios. If a male's estrogen is higher, using zinc daily can help decrease the testosterone being converted into estrogen. Too much estrogen in a male can cause symptoms like low libido, erectile dysfunction, poor cognitive function, and depressive moods.

We've realized that zinc is a naturally occurring substance that can block testosterone conversion to estrogen. You can use zinc when estrogen levels are high to normalize it, which can then reverse some of these abnormalities. What's great about nature is that we have many elements within our natural diet that help control our hormones.

VITAMIN D

Vitamin D, often referred to as the "sunshine vitamin," is a fat-soluble vitamin that has a range of benefits for the human body. Its role extends far beyond its critical function in calcium absorption and bone health. Emerging research has highlighted its potential in mood enhancement, anti-aging, immune system support, and even in boosting testosterone levels and libido.

The mood-improving properties of vitamin D may be linked to its influence on certain neurotransmitters, like serotonin, which are associated with mood regulation. Low levels of vitamin D have been correlated with an increased risk of mood disorders, such as depression. Healthline[58] notes that vitamin D may help reduce depression symptoms and improve overall mood. This connection is particularly compelling given the prevalence of Seasonal Affective Disorder (SAD), a type of depression related to changes in seasons, where reduced sunlight can lead to lower vitamin D levels.

Anti-aging is another area where vitamin D shows promise. The vitamin D receptor (VDR) system plays a role in cellular function and the regulation of inflammation, which are key factors in the aging process. According to a PMC article[59], a well-functioning vitamin D/VDR system may help tackle inflammation and aging. The anti-inflammatory properties of vitamin D are significant, since chronic inflammation is a known contributor to the aging process and various age-related diseases.

The immune-boosting effects of vitamin D are also well documented. Vitamin D receptors are found on immune cells, and the vitamin can

---

58   https://www.healthline.com/health/food-nutrition/benefits-vitamin-d
59   https://www.ncbi.nlm.nih.gov/pmc/articles/PMC10002864/

modulate innate and adaptive immune responses. Mayo Clinic[60] highlights its anti-inflammatory, antioxidant, and neuroprotective properties, which support immune health, muscle function, and brain cell activity. A robust immune system is essential for warding off infections and maintaining overall health.

Lastly, vitamin D's influence on testosterone levels and libido is an area of increasing interest. Testosterone is a hormone that plays a critical role in libido, muscle mass, and energy levels. A study cited by Healthline[61] suggests that vitamin D supplementation might increase testosterone levels.

For men, adequate levels of vitamin D may be particularly beneficial for maintaining healthy testosterone levels, which is a crucial hormone for male sexual desire and libido. A deficiency in vitamin D has been linked to lower testosterone levels, which can negatively affect libido. A study published in the journal "Hormone and Metabolic Research" found that vitamin D supplementation increased testosterone levels, suggesting a direct relationship between vitamin D and male hormone levels[62].

Interestingly, in women, vitamin D may also play a role in sexual health because it may contribute to the regulation of estrogen, which can influence sexual desire. A deficiency in vitamin D has been associated with low estrogen levels, which can result in decreased libido. Research has shown that vitamin D supplementation can improve sexual function in women, including desire, arousal, lubrication, orgasm, and satisfaction[63]. Vitamin D supplementation could be great for you and your partner.

---

60 https://www.mayoclinic.org/drugs-supplements-vitamin-d/art-20363792
61 https://www.healthline.com/health/
    herbs-vitamins-supplements-testosterone-levels-balance
62 https://www.hindawi.com/journals/ije/2018/3720813/
63 https://pubmed.ncbi.nlm.nih.gov/29442353/

EXCESSIVE PORNOGRAPHY

Masturbation can be a healthy part of your life. However, excessive pornography consumption has been linked to various sexual dysfunctions, including decreased sex drive and increased erectile dysfunction during partnered sex. One study that explores this issue is a 2016 article that argues that porn can desensitize sexual response, potentially leading to a decreased interest in real-life sexual encounters and difficulty in achieving erections with a partner. This phenomenon is sometimes referred to as "porn-induced erectile dysfunction" (PIED).

The hypothesis is that overconsumption of pornography may alter the brain's reward system, leading to a need for increased stimulation to achieve the same level of sexual arousal. This can result in difficulties in becoming aroused or maintaining an erection during actual sexual encounters, which do not provide the same level of novelty and intensity as the stimuli found in pornography.

The study suggests that the consistent use of pornography might condition sexual expectations and arousal patterns toward the scenarios depicted in such media. This conditioning can create a disconnect between the user's pornographic experiences and their real-life sexual experiences, potentially leading to dissatisfaction and dysfunction during partnered sex.

It is important to note that the research on this topic is complex and evolving, and not all experts agree on the extent to which pornography use may cause sexual dysfunction. Some argue that the relationship between pornography use and sexual health is not straightforward and can be influenced by various psychological and social factors.

For more detailed information on this study, you can refer to the article on Medical News Today.

CARDIOVASCULAR EXERCISE

The penis is a vascular organ. Having optimized circulatory health will increase blood flow to this vascular organ, meaning you'll have an erection more easily and it will last longer. We put our patients through a comprehensive circulatory assessment so that we can get to the underlying cause and treat our patients as a whole.

WEIGHT TRAINING/RESISTANCE EXERCISE

Lifting weights puts special stress on our muscles. Doing resistance training just twice a week at sufficient intensity can stimulate two hormones that make us feel young: testosterone and human growth hormone (HGH).

Testosterone is the hormone most connected to our libido, so weight training can stimulate sexual desire that can improve erections.

HGH is a hormone that flows most abundantly when we are children. This is the hormone that tells our bones and skin to grow. Eventually, as we become adults, growth hormone subsides or else we would keep growing taller without stopping. However, stimulating a small amount of growth hormone can make you feel young again, rejuvenate your skin and tissues, and even provide a boost in energy.

Compound movements, such as squats, deadlifts, bench presses, push-ups, and pull-ups tend to stimulate more testosterone and HGH production than other exercises. But if you're just getting back into shape or have injuries, you can choose other movements, such as squats and bench presses done on the Smith machine, leg presses, lat pull-downs, and workouts with dumbbells or kettlebells. Start where you are and build up to more challenging exercises with the help of a certified personal trainer.

SLEEP

One of the top things you can do to naturally stimulate your testosterone is better sleep. Better sleep hygiene means no screens before bedtime, going to bed at the same time each night, and waking up at the same time in the morning.

One formula that works well for sleep is MDsleep by MDbio Wellness which was recently found to help 57% reported improved sleep. The study also found that it worked for the majority of study participants after a week of daily use. Learn more here: https://www.mdbiowellness.com/pages/trials#shopify-section-mdbio__trials-summary

The penis is a vascular organ and the more blood flow that we can get to this vascular organ, the better an erection that our patients can have. The way that we optimize this is through physical exercise, our diet, and increasing the blood flow through simple procedures that we have in the office, such as Shockwave Therapy (a.k.a. PulseWave Therapy).

There are five top needs that my patients need to address. One is helping them sleep better at night, whether it's due to frequent urination or just waking up in the middle of the night. Two is sexual optimization, helping them obtain better erections on a more consistent basis. Three is optimizing hormones to make sure that, as we age, we biohack our bodies and stay as young as possible. Four, we check for multiple different types of cancer, prostate cancer, kidney cancer, and testicular cancer on a consistent basis so that none of our patients fall through the cracks. And five, vitamin levels. We check our patients diligently for vitamin levels, such as vitamin B and vitamin D to make sure that their bones are staying healthy as we age.

15. Sexual Rejuvenation for Couples

HETEROSEXUAL COUPLES

ThermiVa Vaginal Rejuvenation and Shockwave Therapy for Male Enhancement

More and more of our heterosexual couples are understanding that their bodies need help in maintaining their youthful exuberance. Most turn to hormone therapy without realizing the added benefits of physical treatments of their genitalia.

When the male partner receives Shockwave Therapy, it not only prevents ED events, it also enhances their performance as they achieve fuller, longer-lasting erections.

The female partner often experiences a tightening of the vagina from just one ThermiVa treatment which also enhances the sensitivity of the clitoris as well as the G-spot usually located inside the vagina behind the pubic bone. They also tend to produce more lubricant, as ThermiVa is an effective treatment for vaginal dryness. I can't tell you how many times our ThermiVa patients have come back to brag about the intensity of their orgasms and how satisfying their sex life had become in their 40s, 50s, and 60s in particular.

Both partners benefit from their partner's treatment. The increased quality and size of the erections offer more potential stimulation of the G-spot for female partners, resulting in a greater chance of pleasurable stimulation and orgasms. The male partner will notice the tighter, more moist condition of their partner's vagina, restoring a teenage playfulness to their sex play. To see those adolescent smiles on my patients' faces as they rediscover the marvels of sex is a priceless experience.

DOUBLE THERMIVA TREATMENTS FOR LESBIAN COUPLES

A couple with two female partners can benefit from a couple's appointment for ThermiVa treatments. Just one treatment can increase collagen production that makes vaginal tissue more supple, elastic, and sensitive to physical stimulation. Vaginal lubrication is increased by the renewed blood flow from the radiofrequency waves that stimulate the blood vessels in the vaginal walls, making for more comfortable and rewarding sexual encounters.

DOUBLE SHOCKWAVE THERAPY TREATMENTS FOR GAY COUPLES

Shockwave therapy can be a shared health regime among gay partners. Not only does it treat ED, but it can also maintain the longevity of healthy erectile function to prevent ED. The penis is filled with blood vessels, so when Shockwave Therapy stimulates new blood vessels to grow and for older vessels to repair themselves, erections become fuller than impaired veins in the penis.

Erectile dysfunction occurs at a rate of about 50% in men in their 50s, 60% in men in their 60s, and 70% in men in their 70s. Shockwave therapy addresses ED at an 80% success rate with my current patients. When adding Shockwave Therapy to a comprehensive treatment plan including medications, lifestyle changes, and penile injections, these numbers improve.

Why wait to become one of the statistics of ED when there are effective treatments to maintain your current sexual performance and enhance it?

BENEFITS OF THERMIVA

What are some of the common reasons we use ThermiVa? The first is vaginal dryness. Many women who suffer from vaginal dryness still want to be on hormones long-term. ThermiVa can change that very easily.

Second, vaginal looseness. Many women want a more youthful appearance but don't want to undergo any surgical procedures. ThermiVa can reverse that quite easily in 30 minutes.

Third, urinary frequency and urgency. A lot of women will develop urinary frequency in their lifetime but don't want to be on medications. ThermiVa can reverse that for many women.

Fourth, recurring urinary tract infections. Many women will start to get recurring urinary tract infections. ThermiVa itself can restore natural vaginal health, and by doing so, prevents bacteria from getting into the urethra as easily, thereby minimizing the number of recurring urinary tract infections.

ThermiVa is also highly effective for orgasms. What do I mean by that? Many women have difficulty achieving climaxes. If they do, it's very muted. ThermiVa, however, can restore the normal blood flow to the clitoris. By doing so, it can allow women to have normal climaxes. Again, many of them will say, "I haven't had one of these since I was in my thirties." It's great to see that it's reversible, and how effective ThermiVa can be for women.

16. The Stud Protocol Challenge

*There is a sexual fountain of youth. It's called the
Stud Protocol.*

The STUD Protocol is a 3-month, focused program that completely
revives your penis, prostate, and libido. This protocol was originally
designed for my patients who were suffering from ED. However, after
the patients recovered their sexual function, they reported that they
are not only having harder, better erections, rather their penis was
actually growing thicker and longer. Their partners also reported
noticing this phenomenon. So I began administering the protocol to
other patients who didn't have ED and quickly discovered the male
enhancement potential of the Stud Protocol. In just 3 months, you
can have a vastly different sexual experience that could potentially
outperform your younger years.

So the Stud Protocol helps both men who are experiencing sexual
performance issues, such as ED, as well as men who want to optimize
the size and reliability of their erections. Remember, you can go beyond
your baseline sexual performance to reach a new level of sexual
prowess. I see the Stud Protocol as the best form of ED prevention.

For those with ED, the goal is to restore a more youthful baseline and
maintain sexual longevity for years to come.

For men that have felt a dip in libido, the Stud Protocol is designed
to supercharge your sex drive and reliability of your erections. I think
of patients in this category as doing ED prevention because they are
ensuring that their hormone levels, nerve, and circulatory health are
optimal.

For men who have frequent erections, but feel inadequate about their penis size, the male enhancement of the Stud Protocol is for you. By receiving several PRP penile injections combined with Shockwave Therapy and the other penile optimization techniques, men are seeing growth in length and girth in their penises. The Stud Protocol keeps on giving as time goes on. So the more you work the program, the more it works for you.

BENEFITS OF THE STUD PROTOCOL

- Increased erection size, hardness, and reliability
- Penile enlargement with repeated treatments
- Increased circulatory health and vascularity in your penis
- Longer sexual endurance before orgasm
- Increase pleasure from rejuvenated penile nerves
- Increased satisfaction in your sexual partner(s)
- Gains in confidence as your Inner Stud emerges

WHAT'S INCLUDED IN THE STUD PROTOCOL

1. Shockwave Therapy
2. PRP Penile Injections +
3. Vacuum Device (Penis Pump)
4. Medications
5. Nitrous oxide
6. Performance boosters
7. A full hormone panel to optimize libido, mood, and energy levels
8. Tony Allemon's Sexual Optimization Customized Diet Plan

Remember, we must treat multiple systems inside the body to be in optimal condition for sex. The Stud Protocol checks all the boxes in the assessments that I do with my patients every day.

17. Clinical Trials at Comprehensive Urology

For the most updated information on our clinical trials and observational studies, visit us at comprehensive-urology.com and click the "Clinical Trials" tab or go directly to https://comprehensive-urology.com/clinical-trials/.

OBSERVATIONAL STUDIES

1. P-Shock: PRP Penile Injections + Shockwave Therapy for ED Treatment and Penis Enlargement
2. Boshox: Botox Penile Injections + Shockwave Therapy for ED Treatment and Penis Enlargement
3. Shockwave Therapy for Prostate Rejuvenation for treatment of BHP, Prostatitis, and ED Treatment

For low-intensity Shockwave Therapy case studies, we are looking at different amplitudes and frequencies and determining which actually results in the best type of erections. We're also studying how modulating the frequency and amplitude can affect results.

For utilization of PRP with low-intensity Shockwave Therapy, we are asking: Can the combination of those two healing powers work better? If so, what's the right frequency? What's the right amplitude? What's the right combination for us to get the best results?

CLINICAL TRIALS

Some of the clinical trials we are performing. Comprehensive Urology includes:

1. TULSA Procedure: The Captain Study is examining TULSA Pro focal therapy for men with prostate cancer. If men have prostate cancer, they no longer have to just have an operation removing the entire prostate or part of the prostate. Now they can have focal therapy using ultrasound-based therapy to target the cancer, specifically outpatient basis. Maximal preservation of quality of life, including sexual function and urinary incontinence. Our clinical study also knows the captain's study. We're looking at the difference between surgery and focal therapy. Most men who have been diagnosed with prostate cancer are relegated to either undergo surgery or radiation, but there are newer modalities looking at focal therapy whereby we're able to identify the location of the prostate cancer and use ultrasound to be able to get rid of it. Now we can provide this as a clinical study for men who otherwise would not have access to focal therapy, whereby the treatment is now covered for them. Under normal circumstances, this can be quite an expensive ordeal, but now through the clinical study, we're able to provide access to so many more men with prostate cancer who are interested in cutting-edge technologies that are highly effective and are able to preserve their normal functionalities, including normal erections.

2. BPH Butterfly treatments: We currently have a clinical study for men with BPH. Many men with BPH can only use medications or undergo surgery, but they're now minimally invasive treatments. Most minimally invasive treatments, though, are irreversible. There's now a reversible modality called the butterfly, whereby we put a small device inside the prostate, which takes about five

minutes and opens up the prosthetic channel so that men can void their bladder normally without the reliance on medications or surgery. The nice thing about this procedure is that it is completely reversible for any reason. If we need to, we can always take it out. It is a highly effective, fantastic therapeutic option for men that don't want to take medication lifelong.

3. Chronic urinary tract infections (UTI's). There are now vaccines that are available to prevent the recurrence of urinary tract infections. Many men and women who get repeated urinary tract infections don't know what to do. We now have a clinical trial at Comprehensive Urology taking a look at the use of vaccinations so that we can immunize the body to fight off infections. You don't have to get repeated infections, again and again, and be on numerous antibiotics.

DR. KIA MICHEL'S CLOSING MESSAGE:

It's never too late to get help with optimizing your sexual performance. But the sooner you ask for help, the more a urologist will be able to offer you. I've had the honor of being a trusted provider to thousands of patients over the past few decades. Seeing them lead more satisfying lives is what drives me as a physician. My hope is that the STUD Protocol and information provided in this book will help you to be more vibrant, feel more confident, and enjoy life to the fullest.

18. References

Chapter 2

Veale, D., et al. (2015). Am I normal? A systematic review and
   construction of nomograms for flaccid and erect penis length
   and circumference in up to 15,521 men. British Journal of
   Urology International, 115(6), 978-986. DOI: 10.1111/bju.13010
   (double check source)
Costa, R. M., et al. (2012). Women Who Prefer Longer Penises
   Are More Likely to Have Vaginal Orgasms (But Not Clitoral
   Orgasms): Implications for an Evolutionary Theory of Vaginal
   Orgasm. The Journal of Sexual Medicine, 9(12), 3079-3088. DOI:
   10.1111/j.1743-6109.2012.02917.x

Chapter 3

https://pubmed.ncbi.nlm.nih.gov/16422843/
https://www.ncbi.nlm.nih.gov/pmc/articles/PMC11035123/
https://www.health.harvard.edu/
   blog/a-new-option-for-orgasm-problems-in-men-201205294804

Chapter 4

https://www.niddk.nih.gov/health-information/urologic-diseases/
   erectile-dysfunction/definition-facts
https://www.ncbi.nlm.nih.gov/pmc/articles/PMC5313296/

https://www.ncbi.nlm.nih.gov/pmc/articles/PMC5313305/
https://www.amjmed.com/article/S0002-9343(06)00689-9/pdf
https://www.ncbi.nlm.nih.gov/pmc/articles/PMC7177870/
https://www.ncbi.nlm.nih.gov/pmc/articles/PMC10318491/
https://www.mayoclinic.org/healthy-lifestyle/mens-health/
    in-depth/kegel-exercises-for-men/art-20045074

Chapter 5
____

https://journals.sagepub.com/doi/10.1177/15579883221087532
https://www.mdpi.com/2072-6651/15/6/382
El-Shaer, W. et al. (2021) 'Intracavernous injection of botox® (50 and
    100 units) for treatment of vasculogenic erectile dysfunction:
    Randomized controlled trial', Andrology, 9(4), pp. 1166–1175.
    doi:10.1111/andr.13010.
https://onlinelibrary.wiley.com/doi/full/10.1111/andr.13010
Abdelrahman, I.F. et al. (2021) 'Safety and efficacy of botulinum
    neurotoxin in the treatment of erectile dysfunction refractory
    to phosphodiesterase inhibitors: Results of a randomized
    controlled trial', Andrology, 10(2), pp. 254–261. doi:10.1111/
    andr.13104
https://onlinelibrary.wiley.com/doi/full/10.1111/andr.13104
https://www.auanet.org/guidelines-and-quality/guidelines/
    erectile-dysfunction-(ed)-guideline#x8064
Shaher, H. et al. (2023) 'Is platelet rich plasma safe and effective in
    treatment of erectile dysfunction? Randomized controlled study',
    Urology, 175, pp. 114–119. doi:10.1016/j.urology.2023.01.028.
https://www.sciencedirect.com/science/article/abs/pii/
    S0090429523000742
Achraf, C., Abdelghani, P.A. and Jihad, P.E. (2022) 'Platelet-rich
    plasma in patients affected with Peyronie's disease', Arab
    Journal of Urology, 21(2), pp. 69–75.
doi:10.1080/2090598x.2022.2135284.

https://www.ncbi.nlm.nih.gov/pmc/articles/PMC10208162/

Geyik, S. (2021) 'Comparison of the efficacy of low-intensity shock wave therapy and its combination with platelet-rich plasma in patients with erectile dysfunction', Andrologia, 53(10). doi:10.1111/and.14197.

https://onlinelibrary.wiley.com/doi/10.1111/and.14197

https://pubmed.ncbi.nlm.nih.gov/8426404/

https://www.mayoclinic.org/tests-procedures/penile-implants/about/pac-20384916

https://www.ncbi.nlm.nih.gov/pmc/articles/PMC10772644/

https://www.medicalnewstoday.com/articles/erectile-dysfunction-and-premature-ejaculation

Geyik, S. (2021) 'Comparison of the efficacy of low-intensity shock wave therapy and

its combination with platelet-rich plasma in patients with erectile dysfunction',

Andrologia, 53(10). doi:10.1111/and.14197.

https://onlinelibrary.wiley.com/doi/10.1111/and.14197

Pastore, A.L. et al. (2014) 'Pelvic floor muscle rehabilitation for patients with lifelong

premature ejaculation: A novel therapeutic approach', Therapeutic Advances in Urology,

6(3), pp. 83–88. doi:10.1177/1756287214523329.

Chapter 6

https://www.urologytimes.com/view/platelet-rich-plasma-appears-safe-feasible-for-peyronie-disease

https://pubmed.ncbi.nlm.nih.gov/35778315/

https://www.sciencedirect.com/science/article/abs/pii/S2050052121000032

Chapter 7

Brandeis, J., Lu, S. and Runels, C. (2024) '(229) a pilot study of a
novel PRP protocol to increase penile length, girth, and function,'
The Journal of Sexual Medicine, 21(Supplement_1). doi:10.1093/
jsxmed/qdae001.219.
https://academic.oup.com/jsm/article/21/Supplement_1/
qdae001.219/7600882
Penile BOTOX injections improve blood flow and other outcomes
in men with moderate to severe erectile dysfunction | HTB | HIV
i-Base
https://i-base.info/htb/45217
https://i-base.info/htb/45217
https://pubmed.ncbi.nlm.nih.gov/34937674/

Chapter 8

https://pubmed.ncbi.nlm.nih.gov/25284738/
https://www.mayoclinic.org/tests-procedures/circumcision/
about/pac-20393550
https://www.ncbi.nlm.nih.gov/pmc/articles/PMC8072165/
https://www.cancer.org/cancer/types/prostate-cancer/about/
key-statistics.html

Chapter 10

https://www.ncbi.nlm.nih.gov/pmc/articles/PMC7327297/
https://www.mayoclinic.org/medical-professionals/
urology/news/high-intensity-focused-ultra-
sound-for-the-treatment-of-prostate-cancer/
mqc-20519431
https://pubmed.ncbi.nlm.nih.gov/33021440/

Chapter 11

https://www.ncbi.nlm.nih.gov/pmc/articles/PMC8908761/
https://www.nejm.org/doi/full/10.1056/NEJM199210223271701
https://www.ncbi.nlm.nih.gov/pmc/articles/PMC10129019/
https://www.ncbi.nlm.nih.gov/pmc/articles/PMC6180381/
https://www.ncbi.nlm.nih.gov/pmc/articles/PMC6373984/

Chapter 14

https://www.healthline.com/health/food-nutrition/
    benefits-vitamin-d
https://www.ncbi.nlm.nih.gov/pmc/articles/PMC10002864/
https://www.mayoclinic.org/drugs-supplements-vitamin-d/
    art-20363792
https://www.healthline.com/health/
    herbs-vitamins-supplements-testosterone-levels-balance
https://www.hindawi.com/journals/ije/2018/3720813/
https://pubmed.ncbi.nlm.nih.gov/29442353/

19. Author Bios

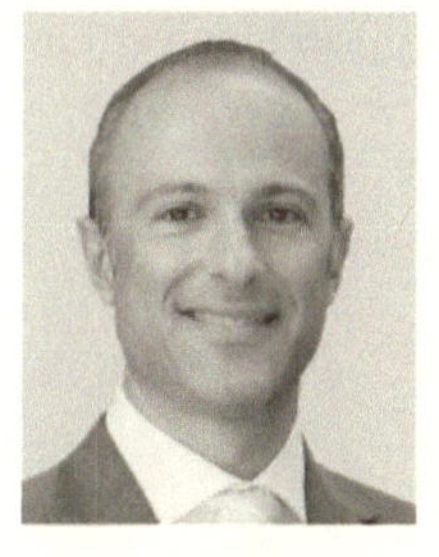

ABOUT KIA MICHEL, MD

With over 25 years of clinical expertise, Kia Michel, MD strives to be the best urologist in Los Angeles by constantly improving our services in our state-of-the-art facility in Beverly Hills. As the founder of Comprehensive Urology, Dr. Michel has solidified his reputation in Los Angeles as a leading prostate cancer expert that specializes in prostate cancer treatment, BPH treatment, robotic surgery, focal therapy for prostate cancer such as HIFU and TULSA, erectile dysfunction treatment, Shockwave Therapy for ED, Botox penile injections, Pyeronie's disease treatment, and testosterone replacement therapy (TRT).

Dr. Michel attended Whitman College in Washington, as a Presidential Scholar. After his undergraduate studies, Dr. Michel completed medical school at the University of Washington School of Medicine in Seattle, where he graduated with honors. He went on to the prestigious University of California, Los Angeles, Department of Urology, where he underwent his residency training. During this time, Dr. Michel was recognized as a National Pfizer Scholar.

Following residency training, Dr. Michel continued to develop his professional skills by completing additional training in urologic cancer surgery as well as becoming a principal investigator on various clinical trials. For his contributions to medicine, Dr. Michel has been recognized by the National Cancer Institute, the National Institute of Health, and the American Urological Association.

Kia Michel MD is also the developer of the STUD Protocol which addresses each aspect of male sexual health to ensure maximum sexual performance. He currently runs observational studies on the latest male enhancement therapies at Comprehensive Urology in Los Angeles.

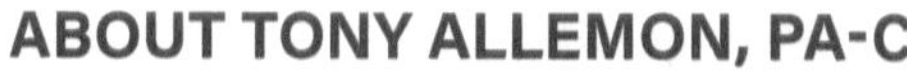

ABOUT TONY ALLEMON, PA-C

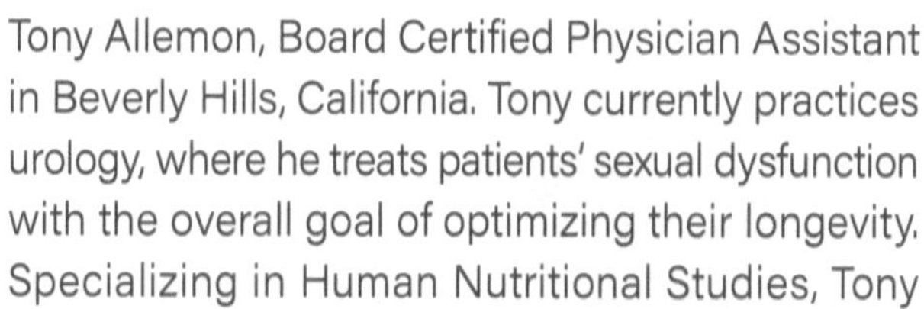

Tony Allemon, Board Certified Physician Assistant in Beverly Hills, California. Tony currently practices urology, where he treats patients' sexual dysfunction with the overall goal of optimizing their longevity. Specializing in Human Nutritional Studies, Tony completed his undergraduate training at Michigan State University before earning his master's degree in Physician Assistant Studies, where he served as class president. Tony has taken his love for nutrition and is the founder/CEO of Tony Allemon Nutrition. In his free time Tony enjoys exercising, playing ice hockey and going to comedy shows with his wife.

Tony Allemon's journey to become a board certified Physician's Assistant began at Michigan State University. He completed his undergraduate studies there, earning a degree in Human Nutrition. Motivated by his dedication to healthy living and his passion for patient care, Tony pursued further education and training. He obtained a master's degree from the University of Toledo, where he not only excelled academically but also stood out as a natural leader. He was nominated to serve as President of his class, demonstrating his strong leadership abilities and commitment to the well-being and success of his peers.

Tony firmly believes in a patient-centered approach, considering it the pinnacle of medical care. He takes pride in dedicating sufficient time and attention to each patient, comprehending their concerns, and crafting treatment plans that cater to their specific needs.

His warm and empathetic nature fosters a strong sense of trust among his patients. This trust allows them to openly discuss their health issues and medical needs, secure in the knowledge that they are in the capable and compassionate hands of a highly astute medical professional.